# SLEEP APNEA

The Complete Guidebook to Understanding the
Symptoms

(The Guide to Eliminating Sleep Disorders Like
Insomnia With Natural Treatment)

**Elias Valentine**

Published By John Kembrey

**Elias Valentine**

*Sleep Apnea: The Complete Guidebook to Understanding the Symptoms (The Guide to Eliminating Sleep Disorders Like Insomnia With Natural Treatment)*

ISBN 978-1-77485-243-9

Legal & Disclaimer

The information contained in this book is not designed to replace or take the place of any form of medicine or professional medical advice. The information in this book has been provided for educational and entertainment purposes only.

The information contained in this book has been compiled from sources deemed reliable, and it is accurate to the best of the Author's knowledge; however, the Author cannot guarantee its accuracy and validity and cannot be held liable for any errors or omissions. Changes are periodically made to this book. You must consult your doctor or get professional medical advice before using any of the suggested remedies, techniques, or information in this book.

Upon using the information contained in this book, you agree to hold harmless the Author from and against any damages, costs, and expenses, including any legal fees potentially resulting from the application of any of the information provided by this guide. This disclaimer applies to any damages or injury caused by the use and application, whether directly or indirectly, of any advice or information presented, whether for breach of contract, tort, negligence, personal injury, criminal intent, or under any other cause of action.

You agree to accept all risks of using the information presented inside this book. You need to consult a professional medical practitioner in order to ensure you are both able and healthy enough to participate in this program.

Table of Contents

# Introduction

This book offers practical steps and strategies for how to deal with insomnia and sleep disorders. It will reveal that the notions of sleep disorder and insomnia is not the identical (more details about the this book). The book will help you find different signs and symptoms of sleep disorders in the initial chapters. You must discover the root cause of sleep problems within your own life. Additionally, you will learn the best way to permanently eliminate sleep disorder by following the advice found in the text.

The book you'll discover the root reasons for insomnia. You will also learn about and how to alter your habits every day, and ways to reduce anxiety, what you should do prior to going to sleep, and what to do to avoid sleeping problems and the best ways to improve your the health of your body and help it rest better, and much more.

# Chapter 1: The Most common types of sleep disorders and Sleeping Disorders

To help you understand sleep disorders and other sleeping issues Here are some of the most frequent kinds:

Insomnia

Insomnia is the inability of a person to sleep. It is usually related to other health issues such as anxiety, stress, and depression. It could be caused by medication you're taking.

The signs and symptoms

You may have insomnia if you're struggling to fall asleep or if you are having trouble sleeping

returning to sleep when you wake up in the middle of the night.

*You wake up from sleep a few times.

*You're sleeping light.

Although you're in a position to rest a bit longer however, you

Still feel tired upon waking up.

*You can't rest without taking sleeping tablets along with other

Supplements.

You are tired and sleepy throughout the day.

Treatment

Doctors aren't able to pinpoint the precise reasons for insomnia. However, a physician would advise you to be aware of your sleeping habits. It is essential to be able to relax before you go to the bed. There are few adjustments that must be made to your life to combat sleepiness. Hypnotherapy can also be a great solution to deal with insomnia.

Sleep Apnea

It is a frequent kind of disorder that affects sleep. Sleep apnea is a condition that occurs when your breathing ceases temporarily during sleep. The pauses in your breathing patterns could result from an obstruction within your airways above.

These occurrences disrupt your sleep and cause you to awake numerous times throughout the time of night. Many sufferers forget about the symptoms, but feel tired during the daytime. They are also unfocused and exhibit low performance at work.

The condition is considered to be serious problem due to the possibility of life-threatening consequences.

The signs and symptoms

Snoring and loud

Sleeping, choking

Gasping during sleep

Feeling exhausted throughout the daytime

Headaches

Breathing shortness

Pains in the chest upon awakening because of an attack of sleep apnea

Treatment

Doctors suggest Continuous Positive Airway Pressure, or CPAP treatment to treat sleep apnea. It is a device shaped like a mask that releases the sensation of a "stream of air" as you sleep.

Sleep apnea may also be due to obesity. Therefore losing weight is essential.

While you're lying down ensure that your head is raised. A side-sleep position can help alleviate moderate to mild sleep apnea.

Snoring

Snoring is a sign that the circulation of air from the nose or mouth to the lungs creates tissues in the throat to vibrate when you sleep. This results in a loud, often loud, sometimes raspy sound. If you or your partner emit loud snoring sounds and you are sleeping, it can be difficult to fall asleep. Snoring could also trigger the development of a serious medical condition such as sleep apnea. Therefore, snoring that is not obvious shouldn't be overlooked.

Common Causes

As you sleep while you sleep, your soft palate (the part of your mouth that sits to the back) as well as your tongue and your throat will relax. If they are too relaxed, they may narrow or completely stop air flow. When you breathe, your salivary glands and Uvula (the tiny tissue that hangs on the surface of the mouth) vibrate, causing sound.

Treatment

The doctors have observed that snoring is more prevalent in males as compared to women, as well as in overweight or obese people. So, their first suggestion for patients is to reduce weight.

If you smoke it is time to stop now.

You can try sleeping sideways instead of lying on your back.

Avoid drinking too much alcohol prior to going to the bed.

Restless Legs Syndrome

Restless Legs Syndrome or RLS is a kind of sleep disorder that is identified by the uncontrollable movements of the legs as well as arms.

The signs and symptoms

The sensations are felt deep inside the legs and accompanied by a strong desire to move them

The sensations are triggered when you're asleep and become more intense in the evening when you're sleeping.

The sensation of being squeezed by needles and pins. Some patients report that their legs get itchy and they feel the urge to scratch at them.

The symptoms can vary from mild to insufferable.

RLS can affect males and females, but it is more prevalent for females. The symptoms may begin to show in childhood.

One of the reasons identified are various chronic diseases like diabetic coma, Parkinson's as well as kidney disease. If you're taking anti-nausea medications and antidepressants, then you are likely to be prone to RLS. It is also believed that pregnancy can cause RLS especially in the last trimester. However, the symptoms typically disappear within the first month following the birth of your child.

Treatment

Although there isn't a known cure for RLS however, doctors suggest a few effective ways to treat the symptoms. Massage and movements can ease the discomfort in the legs. Bathing in hot water is also recommended. Ice packs or heating pads are able to be applied to legs to alleviate the pain. Medicines such as pain relievers and anti-seizure medications can be used.

Narcolepsy

Narcolepsy is a disorder that causes uncontrollable and excessive amount of sleepiness throughout the daytime. This sleep disorder is caused due to the malfunction of the brain's mechanism for sleep and wakefulness to function as it should. The person who suffers from narcolepsy is prone to abrupt "sleep attacks" when working, or when engaged in an argument. This is cause for worry because it could happen at any time, even when driving. This could result in an accident that is fatal.

The signs and symptoms

A sudden feeling of weakness

Feelings of being unable to manage your muscles

You may be able to hear or see things when you're tired

The feeling of beginning to think before you're not

The feeling of being completely immobile or paralyzed when you awake or sleep

Complications

The effects of narcolepsy on sexual libido can be diminished. Some sufferers can even sleep during a sexual encounter because of how abrupt the attacks can be.

If you suffer from narcolepsy, it is not allowed to drive by yourself since sudden episodes could happen while you're driving, and the results could be deadly.

Narcolepsy sufferers are likely to gain weight due to lack of exercise and food cravings.

Treatment

There is no cure for narcolepsy yet, doctors suggest medications and radical lifestyle changes to manage symptoms. The most common prescriptions for doctors are:

The use of stimulants such as armodafinil or modafinil can aid patients in staying awake.

Selective serotonin-reuptake inhibitors, such as fluoxetine and venlafaxine can help reduce signs of sleep disorder as well as hallucinations

Antidepressants

Sodium oxybate helps patients to get an enjoyable night's rest

Lifestyle changes are also necessary:

Make sure you stick to a consistent sleep-wake routine throughout the day especially on weekend days.

You should take short naps throughout the daytime. A 20 minute nap will suffice should you plan it strategically for the daytime.

Stop smoking cigarettes and drinking alcohol drinks.

Ensure regular exercise.

Circadian Rhythm Sleep Disorders

Humans have an internal body clock which regulates the 24-hour cycle of sleep and wake and is called the circadian rhythm. The doctors say that the light of day has a major impact on the circadian rhythms of your body. When the sun rises at dawn, your brain signals to your body that it's time to rise. Then, when it begins to get dark in the evening The brain triggers release of melatonin, which is a naturally occurring hormone that helps promote sleep.

If this rhythm is disturbed, you'll be irritable, sleepy and tired at the least convenient time in the morning. The circadian rhythm is associated with sleep disorders as well as sleep disorders such as insomnia during shifts, and jet time lag. Atypical circadian rhythms have been shown to be a contributing factor to depression and bipolar disorder.

Jet Lag

Jet lag is the temporary disruption of rhythms of the circadian clock when you move between two time zones.

The signs and symptoms

*Fatigue

* Sleepiness during the daytime

*Stomach problems

*Headache

*Insomnia

It is important to note that symptoms may appear in a few days following traveling across 2 time zones. If the travel time is longer, the more severe the symptoms will become. It has been found that symptoms are worse when you fly east compared to traveling west.

Eliminating the symptoms

If you are frequently traveling to work, you must be aware that it takes some time before your body's internal clock is reset. You'll be tired and hungry at odd times. Sleep is often at the most inappropriate moments.

There are several methods to aid you in resetting your body clock before you travel. Travel is definitely planned therefore it is better to gradually alter your sleep schedule between 3 and 4 days prior to your flight in accordance with what time zone is in effect at the area you're traveling to. When the time you get to your location your body clock will be been adjusted to the local time zone, and you will be able to create a sense of normalcy with your sleeping routines.

If you plan to go on long journeys, do not immediately get to bed until the time is at night when you're in the new zone of time. It is best to for the beginning of the trip in nature to ensure the body's clock is adjusted to daylight.

If you are only in the area for a short period it is advised to avoid time-shifting or get up and go to sleep in the morning at your time at home.

Be sure to consume plenty of fluids to keep well-hydrated. Reduce your intake of caffeine and alcohol since they can result in dehydration, which could aggravate the symptoms.

Problems with sleep at night during shifts

Problems with sleep at night in the workplace result when your internal clock isn't in alignment with your work schedule. There are some industries that require 24 hour work hours; consequently, there are workers who work in rotating shifts early morning shifts and even night shifts. The schedule of work changes regularly and can alter the body's clock.

Some people are able to easily adapt to shifting shift schedules, but there are those who have problems. Many shift workers are sleep deprived in comparison to shift workers working during the daytime.

Limiting the Impact

If your schedule changes each month, it will benefit if you were to manage your sleeping-wake cycles naturally. There are strategies to get sleep, even if you have to rest in the daylight hours. If you aren't in control over your shifts it is recommended that you alter your behavior within yourself. In the event that you don't, you may need think about transferring to a different job, but preferably one that doesn't require the possibility of rotating schedules.

If your business is more accommodating in accepting requests for shift changes You might be able to request the shift later as opposed to one earlier from the soon-to-be previous schedule. It is easier for people to shift forward instead of reverse.

Delayed Phase Disorder

A delayed phase condition happens in the event that your body's clock gets delayed. In this case it is when you go to sleep and get up later than most people. If you suffer from this disorder, it can be difficult to perform during regular working hours, such as in a 9-to-5 work schedule.

The problem is not just being a person who wants to be up late. It is more prevalent among teens, and they'll eventually overcome it in a short time. If you are still struggling with the condition getting help from a professional might be the answer.

## Chapter 2: Root Ursaches of Insomnia and Most Sleep Disorders

The information on the symptoms associated with different sleep disorders, that was covered in the previous chapter, will prepare you for this chapter - discussing the root of the issue.

Triggers of insomnia and causes

It is best to start with the most commonly-seen conditionthat is insomnia. It's likely to surprise you to learn that insomnia is one of the most difficult issues also.

Bad Habits

Some people find that the health issue can be attributed to poor habits. In the beginning drinking coffee in the hours prior to the time of bed isn't an ideal idea.Eating too much at dinner could also cause problems sleeping. Constantly sleeping in a poor setting could panic to sleepiness. To be particular, should are asleep when you're in the middle of the night with lights turned on, or when there's still a lot of music playing from the TV it is possible that you will awakening up in the morning exhausted. Don't forget that a deep sleep is essential to feel fully refreshed. However, distractions and interruptions could hinder you from falling asleep deep sleep.

Conditions underpinning the conditions

The bad habits of life are not the sole reason that cause insomnia. The disorder may also be caused by certain health issues. For instance, people with arthritis typically have trouble sleeping during the late at night. Heartburn episodes can also hinder individuals from falling asleep. In simple terms any health issue that is causing pain can pharmaceuticals to insomnia.

Medication

Sometimes, the substances intended to ease discomfort can cause the sleep disorder to manifest. However, this isn't about sedatives. It's about antidepressants and anxiety drugs (which actually combat discomfort, but only those that affect an individual's emotional and psychological aspects). The majority of these medications cause insomnia. as a side effect listed under their effects.

Stress

Unrest in your soul (during your bedtime) is also a cause of insomnia. It's difficult to keep from insomnia if you're a lot of anxious about things. Events that have had an impact on your life (not positive however) can also deprive you of sleep, particularly in the event that you're not yet able to get over the hurt that those events have caused you.

Physiology

Certain biological processes are linked with sleep disorders. For example, pregnancies can cause insomnia. What's the connection between these two conditions? The parents of a child are affected by hormonal changes that can cause hot flashes. Hot flashes are extremely uncomfortable and can result in frequent interruptions to sleep or stop sleeping altogether. This is the case for women who are going through menopausal. The hot flashes experienced during menopausal pregnancy and during menopausal menopausal men similar in that they both result from changes in hormone levels which is why it's not unusual that women experiencing menopausal symptoms also experience insomnia.

Possibility of Apnea

Once the numerous possible causes for insomnia have been explored and discussed, it's time to look at the root causes that cause sleep apnea.

Being overweight is among the most frequent causes of this illness. Being overweight and having excess fat within the body could lung to obstruction of the passages. Central airways, that includes the throat, the nose and the windpipe isn't the only one.

Problems with the brain could be the reason. Because the brain is the primary controller of every aspect of life, including processes which are deemed to be involuntary it can alter breathing. Also, it could stop the respiration system in the event that it is sending incorrect signals (or even if it did not send any signals in the first place).

What are the causes of restless-legs syndrome?

The restless-leg syndrome , on the other hand, isn't solely a brain-related issue It is also associated to nerves.

Damage to the nerve

It's the reason why those who've been injured and suffer from peripheral nerve damage may have random Twitching. But remember that injuries aren't the only reason the nervous system can end with a failure.

## Underlying Conditions

Any medical issue that has negative effects on nerves and the brain may eventually trigger leg jerkiness.People who suffer from kidney disease, for instance are usually prone to periods of leg twitching. Similar to this people who are affected by anemia or diabetes may also end experiencing issues with leg movement.

## Other Triggers

The condition could be caused by certain medications or pregnancy. These risk factors can make this sleep disorder somewhat like the more frequent insomnia.

## The root cause of rarer Sleep Disorders

Science has progressed a lot however, a lot of things remain to be found out in relation to sleep issues. Narcolepsy, for instance, is "unmapped" that simply means that doctors don't know exactly how and the reason why it happens.

Similar to narcolepsy, sleepwalking hasn't been fully understood by scientists. In the simplest sense scientists believe that the disorder is caused by an error in the way sleep-arousal is switched. In a simpler way the sleepwalkers are unable to transition properly from sleep to awake, leaving them stuck in a state between sleep and conscious.

# Chapter 3: The Basic Sleep Mechanisms and the Effects of a poor sleeping routine

The body has a basic requirement for sleeping. In normal conditions the body is able to switch between wakefulness and sleep during an hour. This is called a circadian rhythm. The sleep component includes two kinds of sleep, which are the non-rapid sleep of eye movements (NREM) as well as rapid eye movement sleep (REM).

NREM sleeping is referred to as slow waves. When you are in REM sleep, you are able to activate the capacity to develop memories and learn. This is the condition in where the skeletal muscles of the body are stopped from moving, thereby preventing us from performing our dreams. Imagine what you might be capable of! In the absence of adequate sleep, our hormone balance may be impacted and could be able to pain to chronic illnesses.

For optimal health, a good sleep shouldn't be interrupted in any way, not due to thoughts of thirst, thoughts, or any other physical discomfort. Let's get serious. Is a circadian rhythm ? And what are the consequences of sleep patterns on hormone production?

Circadian Rhythm

The rhythm is an integral aspect of our life. If you take a look around and see that our social activities revolve around the 24-hour rhythm. We get up each day, get ready to get our work done, and then get back to sleep. All this happens within all of the hours.

In the past, it was believed that the internal functions of the body couldn't be affected by external influences from the world. Numerous studies have proved that this completely wrong. It is now clear that our environment inside is always changing and is dependent on external and internal stimuli. That means that what happens all around us may affect our wellbeing.

Sleep patterns are an excellent example of this because light can influence the rhythm of our circadian cycle and the rhythm that follows affects the way that our bodies function. It affects hormone production and release of neurotransmitters that are the main messengers that control the internal workings of our bodies.

The amount of time needed for recovery is different for each individual dependent on the your circadian rhythm, health, age, habits, and health concerns. In general, adults require at least 7-9 hours of sleep over the span of 24 hours. Teenagers need more, about 10 hours. Children's requirements range from 10 to 15 hours, based on their age. [3][1415

"Work to live, but don't work to live."

Unknown

Its effects on the sleep-wake cycle have on hormone production

The human body is a complicated engine. I believe that knowing the mechanisms that govern it helps us take the necessary actions to improve health, happiness and productivity throughout our life. This article is a brief introduction to hormones, some of which you've seen or heard about.

Hormone release is determined by cycles. They are controlled via different triggers. In the first place, hormones are made and released in a strict change that is controlled by a negative feedback system. That is the moment hormone levels rise then the organ ceases releasing or producing new hormones. Additionally, certain hormones trigger different glands to create or release their compounds, and thirdly, the nerve system also plays a role in the process of hormone release.

Sleep is an external factor which definitely affects hormone secretion which is why we must adopt a healthy sleep routine. Numerous hormones are released during the night when we sleep. These hormones have vital functions within the body and show how crucial it is to have a good night's sleep. Certain hormones aid us in getting to sleep, and while we sleep we help in the release of various hormones. Let's look at certain hormones affected by our sleeping habits.

Cortisol

Cortisol is released from the adrenal glands. It is the hormone closely linked to your energy levels. It is recommended that cortisol levels are at a low in the evening and higher during the early morning. This will help us go through the day with an energy level and not to reduce fatigue at night. The secretion of cortisol is determined by our circadian rhythm, so sleep and recovery play key parts in the actions and production of this hormone.

Cortisol secretion becomes haywire when there is stress or sleep deprivation for instance the adrenal glands are exhausted, which can anxious to metabolic issues.

Cortisol is usually released into the body in response to physical or emotional stress. Physical stress may be due to an illness or overwork. Emotional stress could result from life-changing events or even the everyday stresses. Stress can be brought through the loss of a loved one, the loss of employment, and even something as basic like stressing over financial matters or working. Once this hormone is released the body is then prompted to transform amino acids produced by the process of protein metabolism (in other words, out of the muscles) into glucose, which is used for energy. Your body also gets fooled to believe that it is able to store up energy reserves, and consequently that fat builds up in the mid-section of your body. The body is then able to notify the thyroid gland that it needs to stop its functions, which slows down the metabolism of the body.

In order to balance cortisol The body must close down each day. The more stress is present within a person's daily life, the greater the requirement for proper sleep. This is why sleep is so important.

Melatonin

It is the most well-known hormone as far as sleeping is concerned. Melatonin levels increase and decrease over a 24- hour period. The lowest levels occur at noon, and the most intense levels are in the evening as it gets dark outside. Melatonin is the hormone responsible for the feeling of sleepiness. Once we're exposed to light for the second time the production of melatonin is stopped and we cease to feel tired. This hormone is a powerful response to any external stimulus of light.

Melatonin plays a crucial role in the regeneration of muscles and also to reduce inflammation throughout the body.

It is also involved in slowing the process of getting older. When sleep isn't enough inflammation processes are accelerated and muscle growth is slow.

Growth Hormone (GH), Prolactin and Ghrelin

Growth hormone is the main hormone that stimulates our cells in the body to divide and expand. GH is a cycle that occurs every day in which levels are the highest during sleep. Sleep has a powerful influence on the production of growth hormone. This is also the case for prolactin. Together prolactin and growth hormone will burn out the midnight oil literally, by digging into the fat storage in the body while we lie down. This aids in energy production and reduces inflammation.

The stomach produces ghrelin , which produces an appetite-stimulating effect within the body. According to some sleep research, Ghrelin levels are increased when sleep is deprivation. This means that an increase in appetite is correlated with a lack of sleep. When you sleep more the levels of ghrelin are reduced and it becomes much easier to manage your the amount of food you consume. It is also less likely to be overweight.

Thyroid Stimulating Hormone (TSH) and Thyroid Hormone

TSH is the hormone responsible to support the gland of thyroid. It aids in the development of the gland , and regulates the release of thyroid hormones. When the levels of thyroid hormones in the blood get excessively high, the secretion of TSH is cut off.

The thyroid hormone is composed of Thyroxin (T4) as well as triiodothyronine (T3). The principal purpose of this hormone is controlling metabolism of the body.

Sleep plays an important function in the release of TSH which, in turn, affects the release of thyroid hormones. A lack of sleep can have dire negative effects for our bodies. If we don't get enough sleep, the levels of cortisol are lowered and as a result, the adrenal glands get weaker. As a result, the metabolism kicks into high gear through the breakdown of bodily substances. The body will be notified to reduce its metabolism, and the thyroid gland will lose its functions. Hypothyroidism result from a lack of thyroid hormone production. It may result in fatigue as well as weight growth, dry hair the appearance of puffy or swollen eyes as well as thinning eyebrows, thin skin and eyelid swelling and swollen lips.

Hypothyroidism is becoming more commonplace nowadays, however it's certainly not common. If you suspect that your thyroid is deteriorating I would suggest paying close attention to your sleeping patterns before you consider any other supplements. It is of course that a visit with your physician and a blood test are also of paramount importance.

## Leptin and Interleukin-6

Leptin (also known as the satiety hormone) releases by the fat cells within the body after having consumed glucose. The glucose is stored as fat within the fat cells. Leptin is then transported through the nervous system's central region, where it triggers a feeling of feeling full. Another known result of leptin is that its stimulation of the thyroid gland causes it to carry out its tasks. This keeps your body warm and comfortable during your sleep. Research has shown that the levels of leptin decrease in the absence of sleep. This implies that satiety from food isn't achieved at the same speed or in the manner it is normally. Leptin is an essential factor in weight control and appetite. There are at least two functions connected to leptin. First, it traverses the blood-brain-skin barrier and is able to bind to receptors in the center of appetite within the brain, which control brain cells that determine how much you should consume. In addition, it enhances the activity of the sympathetic nerve system, which enables fat tissue to be mobilized to be used as energy. Leptin can also help to reduce inflammation. The body's excessive inflammation could anxious to hypertension and heart illness.

Interleukin-6 (IL-6) is also able to traverse through the blood brain barrier, and it has an impact on temperature of the body. Another aspect that is closely linked to this is the breaking down of fats and tissues. Similar to Leptin, the IL-6 is involved in protecting our immune systems as well as in reducing inflammation.

Sleep deprivation has negative effects upon Leptin and levels of IL-6 within the body. Insufficient sleep can trigger cravings for food and inflammation. This can pharmaceuticals into weight gain, and decrease our immune systems.

As you might have guessed that there is a direct link between sleeping patterns and hormones that are mentioned above. It is vital for the function of the body to get enough sleep every night. It is important to perform a regularly scheduled blood tests to monitor the hormones' response.

Once we have a better understanding of the mechanisms that govern the hormones and body Let's examine the way in which body communicates with brain.

If you can change your mind and make a change, everything else will begin to fall into place.'

-Lao Tzu

The effects of the cycle of sleep and wake on neurotransmitters

Neurotransmitters are chemical messengers that transmit information between neurons of the peripheral and central nervous systems. These chemical signals assist our brains and bodies to function normally. The lack of sleep can have devastating effects on neurotransmitter levels and can affect our memory, cognitive ability and thinking. I think it's just essential to understand neurotransmitters as it is comprehend the functions of hormones. Let's examine the role of some neurotransmitters and how they're in the wake of sleep.

Gamma aminobutyric acid (GABA)

GABA is commonly called a natural chemical valium' is a key component in the balancing of the rhythm that the brain. Insufficient levels of GABA could makeup to depressive symptoms. Research suggests that improper sleeping patterns have adverse consequences on how your body makes use of GABA. In other words, when you don't get enough rest it is possible to experience depression. Other uses associated with GABA are anxiety management, control of muscle relaxation and function. GABA also plays an significant role in the regulation of sleep.

Serotonin

Serotonin is a key player in the circadian rhythm since it changes into the hormone melatonin. Serotonin is also responsible for regulating emotional reactions and alters. A deficiency in serotonin can cause depression. Other uses of serotonin include controlling appetite and is involved in migraine headaches as well as pain. If we don't get enough sleep , we are more prone to depression, depletion of appetite control, and greater susceptibility to pain.

Dopamine

Dopamine is a key function throughout the brain's limbic. It plays a role within the rewards system in the body. Our bodies are able to appreciate certain things as a result of this system of reward, such as eating healthy food or having fun while enjoying activities. It also affects our capacity to remain awake.

Research has shown that the circuits that control dopamine is a neurochemical that we use are affected when we're sleep deprived. Changes in the release of dopamine or its inhibition could nxiety to serious cognitive problems such as addictions, Schizophrenia as well as Parkinson's Disease.

Research has shown that if we do not get adequate sleep, the neurotransmitters we use is seriously impaired. Even 4 hours of lack can trigger changes in the brain's chemical. Each hour of sleep you shed can't be recovered So, rest well and let your brain relax over the next few hours! [7][15][22][23][24][25]

"Early to bed and early rise make an individual wealthy, healthy and smart." -

Benjamin Franklin

## Chapter 4: Limit the the use of Electronic Devices before Bed

Technology has become more and more a aspect to our everyday lives. We are dependent and bonded to technology that we could never be without them. We're always looking at our tablets, phones televisions, laptops, laptops playing video games, and so on. These devices are beneficial as they allow us to stay connected to the world, but they also cause a bit of a distraction in the night when it comes down to. It's normal for users to check their phones when they're in bed, talk to several friends, check email, or play video games. It's possible to fall asleep while you use your phone but awake later in the time to check something. Electronics consume the time that we should be sleeping and making it difficult to get the rest we need. This isn't the only impact they influence our sleeping.

They emit light onto their screens. The light can affect the production process of melatonin that is the hormone that induces sleep. If melatonin levels drop is the inability to sleep , and if we are able to be able to, we are interrupted because of poor transition between cycles. These devices emit blue wavelength light processed by photoreceptors inside the retina. They confuse the brain with the state of the day. The brain has to get ready for bed. Don't just sleep in bed and close your eyes as you drift off to sleep. Younger and older children are the most affected by the blue light emitted by electronic devices. A study conducted on children who used different devices prior to sleeping discovered that they were unable to concentrate throughout the day. This was blamed on less quality sleep when compared to their peers. They also slept less hours, thus not meeting their needs for sleep. Experts suggest that you avoid using any electronic device until an hour prior to going to sleep. This might sound impossible, but remember the information we uncovered in the last chapter. If you're a fan of sleep then you'll go to any lengths to ensure a great night's rest. Do all of your tasks that require a gadget prior to time, but only if it's an emergency. In this regard, take all devices out of your bedroom, including laptops and TVs. Don't bring your mobile phone into the bedroom.

Another reason not to use our devices before going to bed is that they stimulate our brains and keep it active even when we are prepping to sleep. If, for instance, you are working on your emails or play an online game, watch the latest movie or have lengthy conversations with your mobile phone prior to you go to bed, you stimulate the brain and activate it. When you finally go to bed your brain must unwind and move from a state of active to the state of idleness in order to allow you to sleep.

Another reason to eliminate any electronic device from your bedroom is that they can disrupt sleep through their ringing or vibrating. The brain is extremely sensitive to the ringtones we normally hear and even when we are you are asleep you could be awakened whenever this sound plays. It is possible that you don't think about it, however your sleep will be affected. Our aim is to get a good night's rest, not only the the hours we are in bed. Take all of these devices in the bedroom.

According to experts according to experts, kids, teenagers as well as adults, have developed an habit of carrying hands on their devices while in the bed to connect with their friends on social media sites. This habitual association can be unhealthy. The bed is designed to be used for sleep and combining it with other activities can alter the quality of your sleep.

# Chapter 5: The Different Kinds of Sleep Disorders, and What They Signify

A lot of people feel reluctant to visit a doctor or tell coworkers that they have sleep problems. When something is this widespread, it's a shock to see the lengths that people go to conceal their personal struggles.

Consider the situation. If your child that had a sleep disorder What percentage of that do you think it was due to poor behavior? Would you be tolerant of it? The same is true for adults who believe it is their responsibility to be able to be up late at night and check emails or be available throughout the day.

Many people seem to score brownie points when they're capable of responding quickly during office hours, however it is important to note that this may treatment to burning out.

Here's a list situations that are well-known however, they are not often talked about among family and friends.

Sleep Apnea

The term "sleep" refers to sleep. Apnea is a condition that causes breathing to stop and begins, or periods of breathing that are shallow, which happen more frequently than usual. They may last for just a few minutes and are then loud choking sounds and snoring, as well as other disturbing sounds. For children, it could create problems in school because of excessive activity.

It could also trigger complications like strokes, heart attacks, or heart-related failures. The typical age at which it begins is between 55-60 years old.

Sleep Apnea is either an the condition known as obstructive Apnea that is when breathing is disrupted by an obstruction to the flow of air, or central sleep Apnea that is when the regular breathing of an unconscious person ceases to flow. The most prevalent type is the latter, and risks include having a history of family members with the disorder. Other factors are as like having more tonsils that could trigger this. Many people are not aware that they have this condition, only to later be advised by their family members that they disturbed others' sleep at evening.

Insomnia

Insomnia sufferers struggle to sleeping, and their problems aren't consistent. There are times when they find it difficult to fall to sleep, while at other times they may have difficulty to remain asleep after having gone to sleep. They could awake at a young age, being tired and unfocused. This affects the rest of their day and as time goes into the evening, they are exhausted and are unable to complete the majority of physically or mentally demanding tasks.

They may be extremely fatigued and sleepy. People who suffer from insomnia can even be unhappy and suffer from mood fluctuation. The condition can cause anxiety and could generations to depression, schizophrenia and various other conditions.

If an individual's performance at work or everyday functioning starts to decline, insomnia could be the reason. What's the reason for insomnia? It could result from a variety of diverse causes, and it could be a temporary stress-related condition. In most cases insomnia is a sign of an untreated health issue.

Imagine one of your children or siblings is suffering from an illness and falling asleep could result in not experiencing vital changes to their overall health. Other causes could be sleeping in a space that is loud or in a kind of mattress or bed that isn't firm enough or soft, or too high, etc.

Another issue could be that you're not exercising enough and if you suddenly have to be you to drive and walking, whereas before it was walking, your sleeping pattern and routine may be out of in sync. Another risk is using alcohol or drugs, particularly those with high alert levels such as cocaine or MDMA.

One possible psychological cause could have to do with nightmares resulting from the trauma of a past experience. Recurrent nightmares must be addressed as soon as it is.

Particularly frustrating is when you shell out $60 for an hour's worth of time and get the same guidance you'd receive from a book for $7!

Other causes could be chronic pain that one accepts in the daytime however, the pain becomes difficult to ignore at night, especially when they're by themselves in darkness.

Women who are experiencing menopausal symptoms and are experiencing hormonal changes may also experience interruptions of sleep. Insomnia could be an indication of Alzheimer's disease because the early signs often signal disturbances of the brain.

Research has also shown that insomnia could be due to too much screen time' or use of electronic devices prior to going to bed. This is particularly problematic for children and teens.

They can be awake all night and keep in touch with friends, but they are not regulating how much time they spend on the internet.

In the end, teens are rebels and often hide their tablets or phones within their beds or in their bedroom.

The use of antidepressants excessively early (or excessively late) during the day may result in sleep disturbances. This could makeup to low concentration at work or school as well as a lack of coordination in body movements, and other incidents.

Sleepiness can be temporary or continuous and primary insomnia can be an isolated issue, while secondary insomnia could be a sign of an additional issue. It is also defined by the degree to which it affects an individual and the impact it has on their sleep patterns.

Therefore, treating it is just one aspect of the bigger picture Another issue is determining the kind of insomnia the sufferer has.

Certain well-studied studies show that blinds with blackouts or sleeping without an easily reachable mobile phone or bathing prior to bed, and having a sense of a regular nighttime routine can help greatly.

Narcolepsy

It's a chronic sleep disorder that is characterised by an overwhelming, sudden fatigue and sleep attacks. The sufferers of this disorder have a difficult time to stay awake whatever they're up to. It could cause significant disruptions to your daily routines.

People can fall asleep without warning, at any time even in conversation. After a while, even if you've been feeling refreshed and awake but you feel tired.

There is also a decrease in alertness, as well as drowsiness during the course of your day. It's difficult to focus and this makes it difficult for any person to focus.

There could also be an abrupt decrease in muscles that is associated with it that could cause speech slurring and weaker muscles.

It's an uncontrollable disorder Some people suffer this effect more intensely than others. Some episodes every day, when they laugh or experience intense emotions.

Hypersomnia

Hypersomnia is another term, which is a term used to describe a prolonged period that is spent in bed, or greater levels of sleepiness throughout the period of the day. It is a condition where a person is finding it difficult to stay awake.

This can be as a result from not getting a proper night's sleep, being overweight, taking drugs alcohol, or the result of an injury to the head. A few studies have demonstrated that genetics play a major factor in the development of hypersomnia and tranquilizers can make the condition more severe.

Jet Lag

It is also known as the "time zone change syndrome, also known as desynchronosis. It is most common when people frequently travel between time zones or when sleep is disturbed due to shift work.

It's also a disorder of the circadian rhythm that occurs when there is an interruption in the internal clock.

The symptoms are more severe traveling towards the East in comparison to travel towards the West.

Jet lag could be the main reason for sleepiness, irritability and headaches when flying. Also, it is less affecting children than it does adults.

Restless Leg Syndrome

This condition, often referred to by its abbreviated name (RLS) is the predominant requirement for movement of the legs in particular when someone is sitting or lying still. You can see (or perhaps you have experienced from experience), Restless Leg Syndrome can seriously affect sleep patterns.

It isn't clear the root of the issue however, the absence of dopamine and iron deficiency lead to the continuous movement of the legs which leads to a lack sleep and the much-needed relaxation for your body.

Certain prescribed medicines can cause dizzy spells. However, more alternative treatments like yoga and dopamine boosting supplements could be more advantageous. Focusing on the health of your gut can also help. If you suffer from RLS you are likely to have the symptoms listed below all too well.

In bed there is a strong urge or even a sharp feeling that is stinging and pushes that you move your legs.

When you finally take a step out of bed and move around your steps, the relief won't last long, and it's long before you must get up and move again. The condition affects 10 percentage of American people.

Perhaps a better option for this neurosensory condition is to look into supplements and natural cures. Supplements and remedies can temporarily ease the pain however, they should help people to rest in the night.

## Chapter 6: How Does Your Diet Affect Your Sleep?

We must know what our bodies do to get us to sleep, before we can determine what foods work best to ensure a good sleep. There are four primary minerals that help sleep. Tryptophan Magnesium and Magnesium are the most important, along with Calcium B6 and Magnesium. There is a way to consume these minerals as pills, though the most effective option is to add them into your diet.

Here are the most nutritious food items to include in your diet to meet the requirements of all the essential minerals.

1)Tryptophan The substance is an amino acid which stimulates your pineal gland to release Melatonin. As the time for bed approaches, your body's natural release of Melatonin into the bloodstream to aid in preparing you for sleep.

The organic meats include lamb liver, chicken, beef pork, venison, and lamb.

* Seafood: Mackerel, tuna, shrimp, halibut, herring, crab, lobster.

"Dairy products": yogurt cream, cheese, milk.

* Fresh fruit: Avocados, cherries, mango, pineapple, oranges, mandarins, bananas, kiwi.

* Fresh vegetables: All green vegetables, spinach, parsnips, mushrooms.

• Nuts: Tiny portions of high-fat nuts, such as almonds, peanuts, and cashews.

* Whole grain: Bulgur Barley, red Rice corn, oats, and corn.

* Legumes Chickpeas, cannellini beans Fava beans French legumes, green beans, lentils beans, sweet snappea.

2.) Magnesium organic sedative aids in relaxing your body because it regulates the level of adrenaline. The level of hydration is improved by a healthy amount of magnesium, and muscles are able to relax. Here are the food items that can help you increase your magnesium levels:

* Fish: Cod, Salmon herring, mackerel.

* Legumes small red bean, kidney beans, frijol bola de roja, yellow and green peas alfalfa.

* Vegetables with dark leaves: Kale and mustard leaves and broccoli. the chard, arugula, collard greens.

* Bananas

* Dairy products with low-fat content such as cottage cheese and yogurt.

* Grains

* Dried fruits: Raisins dates, cranberries, pineapple Apricots, raisins.

3.) Calcium: We're well aware of the necessity for calcium to strengthen bones and teeth However, did you know it could also aid sleep? Calcium helps your brain process tryptophan and create melatonin, which aids in sleep. Additionally, it regulates blood pressure. enhances the expansion and contraction of muscles.

The calcium-rich foods listed here can aid in preventing insomnia:

* Chinese cabbage: Bok choy, Pak Choy.

* Soy products: Tofu, soybean, soymilk.

* Okra

• Cruciferous green leafy leaves

* Green leaves that are edible Dandelion, Red Clover watercress, chickweed plantain.

* oily fish anchovies herring, tuna, herring salmon.

4.) B6: Your body requires serotonin. It is a neurotransmitter that helps to promote sleep and regulates the cycle of sleep. Vitamin B6 assists the brain convert a small amount tryptophan to serotonin. These foods will help to keep a healthy amount of B6 in your daily diet:

"Organic" meats: Steak chicken, beef, venison Mutton, pork, lamb.

* Seafood: Swordfish, lobster, cod, halibut, mussels, salmon.

* Dried fruits

* Avocados

The Cruciferous Leafy Greens include Kale mustard green and broccoli.

* Chickpeas

* Garlic

* Tuna

* Spinach

What drinks can help improve your sleep patterns?

Minerals aren't just found in food , but they are also present in drinks. Drinking a drink at night can fit perfectly into your routine at night and increase the mineral levels of your body. Drinking any of the following drinks before going to bed will prepare your body to be ready for sleep and also increasing the mineral levels of your body.

Warm milk: Rich in tryptophan and calcium; it is the best way to stimulate our body's own natural "sleepy" hormone, melatonin.

* Cocoa If warm milk isn't enough to buoy your boat, try cocoa. The Mayans were among those who first drank cocoa. They cooked it with roast cacao beans and hot water and spices.

It is a chamomile-based tea. absence of caffeine and its mild taste of chamomile makes it excellent for relaxing the body and mind. It eases tension and helps to settle stomachs, making it the ideal way to relax before the night.

• Passionfruit tea A delicate drink that calms the nerves The tea of passionfruit is loaded with vitamins and minerals.

* Valerian tea Constructed using essential oils extracted from the root of valerian plants,. This herbal tea is known to promote healthy sleep and reduces stress.

This tea is particularly beneficial for women who suffer from menstrual issues.

* Juice of tart cherries The best source of melatonin, a natural chemical.

If you're looking add sweetness to any of these drinks, use honey instead of refined sugar. You can also add the natural sweetener.

Drinks and food to avoid

* Alcohol: Many think that drinking a drink at night will aid in sleep, however in reality, it can disrupt your sleep patterns.

* Caffeine: Stay clear of any caffeine after 2pm to assist you in sleeping. There are many unexpected sources of caffeine, here are a few products that which you don't know contain caffeine: Energy drinks pain relievers including diet and regular chocolates, sodas, as well as decaf and mesquite coffees. Decaf drinks are not always caffeine-free, so make sure you check the caffeine levels of these items.

Foods that are fast: Fast food is more difficult to process than healthy meals. If you have food sitting in your stomach, it will make it difficult to relax properly.

* Foods high in fat

* Foods with a kick

* Refined carbs: Bread white rice, cakes, cookies, cakes crackers, pie, and even candy.

* Pasta

* Nicotine

If you're in need of an energy boost before bed There are a few of fantastic recipes that are nutritious and won't disturb your sleep. Check out these healthy snack options to boost your mood prior to you go to bed.

Banana peanut bagel

The tryptophan-rich fruit and peanut butter with magnesium can help relax muscles and act to act as an eminent relaxant your nervous system.

Ingredients

1 banana that is overripe

1/2 of a whole bagel for a meal

1 Tbsp natural peanut butter with a crunchy texture.

Mash with the banana inside the bowl. Toast the bagel, then spread on it peanut butter. Serve with the banana and serve.

Green fruit salad

Serves four people.

Ingredients

Two cups honeydew Melon

1/2 cup of grapes that are seedless

1/2 cup peeled, ripe Kiwi fruit cut in quarters

Half a cup of yogurt

A splash of lime juice

2 Tbsp fresh mint

Combine the fruits and store up to 4 hours prior serving. Serve with lime juice and yogurt and garnish with mint leaves.

Almond butter and smoothie with bananas

Ingredients

1 . Small frozen Banana

1 cup almond milk 1 cup almond

1 tablespoon honey

1/2 1 tsp ground cinnamon

Blend all the ingredients together in a blender, and blend until smooth. Ice cubes are able to be added to chill the smoothie , if needed.

As with all foods, these meals are best consumed at least one hour prior to going to bed.

# Chapter 7: Background And Facts About Insomnia

What effect does Insomnia affect our health?

Sleep is not a brand new idea to us. In fact sleep has been essential for both animals and humans in order to live. For us, it's much more essential. There are references to sleep throughout the ages. The Bible as well as the Babylonian Talmud both mention sleep often. Sleep problems are frequently described in these works too. In some of the written works writers use terms to express their patterns of sleep. These seem a lot similar to the narcolepsy.

We are all aware that sleep disorders aren't new, but the advancement of technology makes it much easier to identify these and manage them. Research into sleep began around 1800. According to reports, sleep scientist Richard Caton, was one of the first people to conduct studies on animals that were small when they were asleep. They later helped him understand the various stages in our cycles of sleep. A few years after the work Caton carried out, medical texts first discussed Narcolepsy as a condition. It was not that until after the turn of the century when more research was conducted regarding sleep disorders and more of them were classified and named.

Insomnia is the most commonly reported sleep disorder, it's typically temporary and accounts for around 30% of the people who have it are diagnosed. There is no way to know exactly when it was diagnosed, but it's obvious that people weren't receiving enough sleep, and this was likely taking place for a long time as well.

The term "narcolepsy" was used all way back to the earliest texts to the fifteenth century. In 1937, non-REM sleep disorders were discovered. Alfred Loomis began to do more research on sleep disorders and sleepwalkers. There's been a lot of research conducted on the different sleep disorders, and as you've seen there isn't a known cure for a lot of these. In the meantime, as we dig into these conditions, here are a few of the most fascinating information regarding insomnia.

Information about Insomnia

The majority of us do not have enough sleep but does that suggest that we suffer from insomnia? It's not necessarily the case however, if you do experience insomnia it'll be short-lived unless there's a medical condition that's associated with it. The consequences of sleeping less can be a major problem. The quality of our work and relationships will be affected. There are numerous facts about insomnia that could help determine the reason you suffer from it.

There have been a few amount of cases of insomnia in which the sufferer died. This kind of insomnia is known as Familial Fatal Insomnia and it is uncommon, yet it could cause someone to never sleep. This could connected to death. Family Fatal insomnia can cause the person sleeping to not get enough rest to keep their brain functioning properly. This causes the loss of mental function and coordination. This is a genetic type of insomnia. Death could occur between eight to 75 months following the diagnosis.

The signs and symptoms that are a sign of Familial Fatal insomnia may begin with small issues getting to sleep and getting to sleep. Sometimes, the sleeper may be able to feel spasms while asleep. The body can be moving a lot while they the night, with punching and kicking during sleeping. In the near future, they'll start to feel a loss of coordination, and their mental functions gradually begin to decline. The blood pressure and heart rate can also rise. As of now, there are no treatments available however, doctors are able in finding ways to assist those suffering from insomnia sleep as much as they can.

Sleep disorders like insomnia which can result in more than just the loss of energy and sleep. It can also trigger drinking and drug abuse. People who aren't sleeping tend to use alcohol or substances that cause depression, to aid in finding sleeping. This is the reason why many sufferers begin to become dependent of these drugs.

Impacts of Sleeping Disorders on Health

There are millions who are suffering from insomnia. The medical profession often ignores it however, for those who suffer from insomnia at night it can truly impact both the body and mind. The majority of us need seven to eight hours of rest each night to be able to function. If that is interrupted by any means, we'll begin to feel the effects almost immediately. The lack of sleep make us feel drowsy however, it could trigger our emotions to get worse. Here are some of the consequences that a lack of sleep could affect our lives.

A lack of sleep can treatment to accidents. It is interesting to note that historians frequently attribute sleep deprivation to numerous disasters like Three Mile Island, the Exxon Valdez oil spill as well as The Chernobyl explosion. What did sleep deprivation have in connection with the disasters? Three Mile Island nuclear plant is located in Pennsylvania. The cause of this was sleep deprivation. for the disaster as the employees were sleeping less sleep and didn't detect any small defects in the reactor. They were not aware the leak of coolant and this led to an unintended chain reaction within the reactor. Because they did not see what was going on, since they were consumed by exhaustion and exhausted, the reactor was overheating. Luckily, there were just minor injuries resulting from this incident and there were no fatalities.

It is believed that the Exxon Valdez oil spill is blamed on sleep deprivation since Captain of the ship not had much sleep following an evening of drinking. The captain was awake for nearly 18 hours.

The entire crew was experiencing fatigue, and overwhelmed.

Finally, Chernobyl has been blamed for the deprivation of sleep. The employees of the plant worked for at least 12 hours per day due to having to follow strict guidelines. As investigators investigated the cause of the accident they blamed it on stress of the employees.

Sleep deprivation is extremely dangerous when it involves driving too. Tiredness can affect your reaction speed and lead you to crash your vehicle when you fall asleep behind the steering wheel. Employees who are required to endure long hours at work are tired to the max and tend to be more prone to accidents on the job.

Health issues could arise in the event that you do not get enough sleep. Heart ailments as well as high blood pressure strokes, and diabetes could all result from insomnia. Together with these ailments insomnia can stifle the sex urge. Sleeping less reduces the libido of your partner and decreases interest in sexual intimacy in general. With a lack of energy both genders might be more focused on sleeping than their partners.

Sleep deprivation is frequently related to obesity, too. The less sleep you're getting in the night could be the reason you're over weight. Sleep deprivation is usually linked to having lower quantities of leptin. Leptin is a hormone that reduces appetite, and is released while you sleep. If you don't get enough sleep leptin production is reduced. This makes you constantly hungry. It is well known that eating too much can lung to weight gain, so these two factors are inextricably linked.

As you can see, sleep and insomnia can lead to disasters in our lives as well as our world. Consider how Chernobyl could have been a more peaceful place to live if the meltdown didn't happen and if workers had a bit more rest. It's pretty absurd to think that sleep deprivation could cause such huge issues. There is a way to manage insomnia using organic methods, and these techniques provide us with the hope that we will not suffer many more problems since we'll all get the proper amount of rest each night.

# Chapter 8: Sleep and Physical Health

The causes of insomnia could be behavioral, mental physical, or environmental. Although it is simple to classify causes, they mix in a way that makes it difficult to pinpoint the cause. However, there are crucial physical causes of insomnia that require immediate attention and treatment.

Allergy Symptoms

The changes in climate, seasonality or heredity may be the reason of insomnia. For instance, respiratory disorders such as Asthma or difficulty breathing due to dust in the air, or perhaps an small difficulty in breathing due to dust.

Allergies can be unpredictable as they are prone to be triggered to any degree.

The Pain

A single of the frequent factors that contribute to insomnia are physical is chronic or mild such as headache jaw pain, neck pain, back pain muscular pain, arthritis and weakening of the constitution that can cause frequent stomach spasms, etc.

Women with insomnia

Changes in hormones during the premenstrual as well as postmenstrual, early or late pregnancy, post-menopausal or pre-menopausal can cause physical discomfort. Women sleep less well than men, and these issues can only increase the physical stress they experience.

But, it is not conclusive that this proves that men are less susceptible to sleep disorders.

Exercise and nutrition

What you consume and drink directly affects the quality of your sleep. The consumption in the form of Caffeine and Alcohol can have a negative impact on sleep, as they are stimulants. The absence of exercise can lead to a decrease in vitality within your body. This causes physical exhaustion. This affects the sleep cycle.

Medication

Anti-depressants are the main cause of insomnia. There are many over the counter medications for minor health issues like cough and cold can be an important factor in the cause of insomnia. Heart medication, Asthma medications, Anti-Smoking medications are the main factors which can cause the environment to be ruined for an ideal sleeping.

Other Obstructions

Thyroid, Digestive Inflammation, Chronic Fatigue syndrome, Acid Reflux, Bowl Syndrome, Gastric infections etc.

Physical effects of sleep absence

As the body is unable to maintain vigor and energy due to sleepiness, it can have an immediate impact on your overall health and can turn a mild bout that you have experienced into a chronic

Eye Bags, Dark Circles as well as Eye Bags If you are able to leave your body wanting to rest It reflects on the eye area that need rest from strain.

Uncontrolled pulse

Greater risk of Coronary Heart Diseases

Prostate cancer risk due to working late hours

High blood pressure

Strokes

Diabetes

Poor motor skills impact our driving skills and work performance, etc.

Significant genetic changes as a result of the long-term and continuous loss of sleep e.g. overweight (due to a slowed Glucose metabolism) and hypertension

Major dip in sex drive due to depleted energy levels

The process of aging accelerates -tiredness which manifests as wrinkles that appear on the face

Risk of death increases due to an excessive load on vital organs

A slow healing procedure (wounds require much longer to heal because of a weak immune system)

Indulgence in heavy drugs can be viewed as a cause and effect. The use of medications to restore lost sleep can create an endless cycle in which the person who is the savior becomes the victim.

Every issue can be solved; you must discover it and then cement it by focusing, discipline and a sense of calm.

# Chapter 9: Measures to Remedy Physical

Sleeplessness is among the most frequent conditions that can make your day-to-day activities unusable. Adults require seven to 8 hours of sleep to boost their productivity. Sometimes, changing the routines that cause sleeplessness can eliminate sleeplessness completely. It could take several days before your body can adjust adjusted to the change however, once you have done then you'll sleep more comfortably.

Avoid Caffeine

Caffeinated drinks are Diuretics which disrupt sleep.

Avoid Alcohol Beverages

Do not drink alcohol at night. Although alcohol can cause you to feel sleepy, it then can affect the quality of sleep.

Avoid Nicotine

Stop smoking cigarettes or stay clear of smoking at night because nicotine can cause a buzz and interferes with sleep.

Meditation

A regular practice of meditation can help promote harmony between the conscious and sub-conscious. The practice of slow breathing and mindfulness enhances the harmony of the seven Chakras within our bodies.

Hypnosis

It causes Physiological changes and helps in calming the blood pressure as well as the fluctuating patterns of the brain. The most well-known methods of hypnosis is Aroma Therapy. Aromatherapy oils that smell sweet like Chamomile, Ylang Ylang and Lavender etc . neutralize body's temperature when utilized in a bath that is warm.

Yoga exercises

Closely linked to meditation and its origins from Indian Philosophy. This is spiritual connection between the body and mind. It brings an increase in flexibility and suppleness to the body, as well as extreme positive thoughts. A thirty minute daily practice can result in significant improvement in sleep quality.

Herbal remedies

It is based on two pillars: Ayurveda as well as Neuropathy (India's traditional system of natural of treatment)

By using eye masks and earplugs

Sleeping position in the right

Management of weight

Diet

Have breakfast as a King by consuming a lot of Fiber and Calcium intake, as well as Vitamin. This will help reduce cravings and untimely eating habits, while keeping your blood sugar in check. Make sure to include dairy products. Eat food items which contain Lecithin which is a potent sources of Vitamin B (egg yolks and grape juice, cabbage, etc.). It has beneficial effects in improving sleep and brain function. Do not use sugar substitutes made of synthetics. Avoid eating junk food (which is high in Trans Fats).

Take warm milk to bed at night.

The amino acids present in milk can induce sleep that produce serotonin, a brain transmitter that improves the quality of sleep.

Other measures

Do not watch TV or Computer at night.

Keep the lighting in the room low and calming.

Make sure you have a mattress that is comfortable for the body.

Do not drink too much fluids before bed (will determined to frequent trips to the bathroom, thereby disrupting your sleep cycle)

Introduce carbohydrate-rich meals at night which boosts the proportion of tryptophan, an inducer of drowsiness.

Introduce the hormone melatonin (naturally produced hormone that is believed as a regulator of the sleep cycle of the brain) into your diet. It is recommended to take it at least two hours prior to bedtime.

# Chapter 10: Mindfulness: Training the Brain to Find Its Peace

When people talk about fitness it is usually about the body. Exercise is known to have benefits for the body, but there are also mental benefits to be enjoyed too. Apart from the physical advantages of physical exercise, there are also brain-training exercises to keep the mind alert and flexible for the duration of throughout the day. From the mobile app, "Lumosity" to simple crossword puzzles , there are options to keep your brain active in a way that is learning.All of these activities can help keep your mind sharp. They will also assist you in learning to connect with your mind to help you calm yourself when you need to.

We were used to thinking that mental declines, including the ones that caused weaker memory, less hand/eye coordination, and other tasks occurred at the end of our lives. People joke that they are "senior moments" but new research shows that these declines occur sooner in our lives than what we imagine. Researchers in one study found that the first of these declines occurs around the time of the 20s, and that the declines persist at the rate of around 15 percent every 15 years after. The same study also revealed the link between a happy and healthy brain and the capacity to attain a calm state more quickly.

Richard Carmona, writing in his most recent book,"The Canyon Ranch's 30-Days to a Healthier Brain is adamant about the relationship between the body, mind, and spirit seriously. He adds another element to the mix. Carmona believes that eating a balanced diet is crucial for the health of your body and brain in addition.

There's a line to be observed here. A functioning brain may be a healthy and happy brain, but what happens at night when you'd like to go to sleep but the thoughts will never stop from coming? This is the point where brain training is required. The way you speak to yourself and the way you behave with your mind can dramatically change.But first, here are one of the most obvious ways to sleep better and a better mind:

Make sure to dim your bedroom as much as you can. Even the smallest light source from the phone could disrupt sleeping patterns and prevent you from getting an energizing and restful night.

Remove all electronics from the room, including your television and laptop. If you do have to have your mobile device in the bedroom try to keep it away from your head to ensure that it does not cause any problems. I'll explain more about electronics in one second.

It is important to cool the space. The body's temperature should decrease just a bit to help you get a better sleep. There isn't a perfect temperature- but you can try for at least a few degrees lower than the daytime temperature.

Then, we'll return to electronic components and the troubles they create. The place you live in is an EMF hotspot and you weren't aware of this. Before you panic, let me explain. EMF refers to electromagnetic field, and the earth is actually an EMF hotbed by itself. However, the distinction between earth's electromagnetic pull and human-made EMFs lies in the frequency of oscillation as well as the closeness the human body. The EMFs originate from the earth and are separated from us by walls and floors in the walls of our homes.The EMFs in our homes are present, typically within the walls, right next to our mattresses. The more brittle the walls, or the more brittle the insulation, the more close it is that you're to EMF within the space. While you cannot completely stay away from the wiring inside your house, you are able to alter the EMF inside your bedroom better or worse depending on what you allow into it. The more electronic devices you have, the more powerful the EMF increases.

EMFs influence sleeping in two distinct ways. It first activates the brain off. Your brain activity is measured by certain frequencies , many of which are dependent on oscillations. Your brain could slow down to around 2 Hz while you sleep, which is a very slow oscillation. The typical home EMF can operate between 50-60 Hz, which could bring your brain to a higher level , or even stop you from falling into sleep at all in the first place.

Second, EMFs may interfere with the production of melatonin by the brain. Melatonin is a hormone which is responsible for the majority of sleep and relaxation. It is possible to supplement with it, but many people discover that it does not perform regularly or it functions in a way that is too effective. A few people have reported having vivid and odd dreams while taking Melatonin supplementation. It is best to go to bed in a natural manner. The aim is to remove as many electronic gadgets in the bedroom as you can. If you have the money then there are other alarm clocks that eliminate the necessity for your cell phone to be placed on the bedside table. If you can't be this far away from it, think about putting the phone in an area that is drawer, at a minimum. The TV should not be placed in your bedroom as when you are undergoing brain training, you will be using your bed only for two things: sleeping and sexy.

Here are some exercises that will assist you in training your brain to achieve more deeply and restful sleep:

Exercise One: Obtain Success Through Association

If you were to drop a hammer onto your foot each day for one month, you'd be able to associate the sight of a hammer to the sudden pain in your feet. If you are adamant about your bed as well as your bedroom with sleeping and a quiet night and sleep, the sight will make you feel calm and tired.To achieve this it is your goal to establish a routine for bedtime which you adhere to every night as closely as you can until your brain is able to recognize that these movements signal sleep and shuts off without a struggle. The ritual you choose to follow may be as easy as cleaning your face, brushing your teeth, and then putting on pajamas or more complicated. For example, I perform a very gentle yoga routine and then I take a hot bath prior to going to bed. For some who exercise are done close to bedtime may cause heartbeats to rise to a high level, however for me, it's effective. Create your own personal ritual and feel and feel free to add your own elements. A warm cup of milk or hot chocolate could be a good alternative. The act of reading a chapter in the book in a light illumination can be equally effective.

Exercise Two: Use Verbal Cues and Positive Self-Talk to establish Sleep Time

Have you ever awakened in the middle of the night then thought to yourself "I am not going back to sleep!" Did you fall into a deep sleep after or did you trick yourself into shifting and tossing? What you say to yourself can determine whether you perform or fail in whatever you're trying to do. Stop focusing on negatives now and focus on reframing the situation. You've woken up, and now you're going to tell yourself "I am going for a bathroom. I'm going to grab an excellent glass of water, and then to go back to bed and go into sleep."

However, this positive conversation should begin before you awake in the late at night. You can say things like "I am heading to bed, and I'll soon fall asleep" in place of "I will never fall to sleep this evening." In the event that you find yourself slipping back into negative thoughts be aware of the things you're saying. Are there any themes that are consistent? Is there something you are able to refer to over and over? If so then you need to address that problem as soon as is possible. After that, you can reframe the issue as one that can be solved when you talk to yourself about sleeping.

Exercise Three: Set up an Worry and Stress Station

Stress and worry are aspect of our lives and unfortunately there isn't a single way to eliminate these. However, you can educate yourself to be better at handling them particularly when it comes to sleeping better. The effort to avoid stress and everything you're concerned about is likely to cause you to think about the issues more often when you are in less control over your thoughts. You're trying to go off to sleep , but your brain is always thinking about a bill that is due and a presentation you will deliver in a couple of days. And now, you can't sleep. What is the best thing to do?

The first thing you should do is recognize the issues and make a clear strategy for how you'll take care of the issues. The plan should contain the timeframe. Once you've set the strategy, you will be able to tell yourself that there's no way to make amends to fix it tonight, and it's time to go to bed. You can, for instance, keep in mind that this debt is not due until the morning, and you'll be able to pay it later. The presentation will not last only a few days. You can meet the challenge on the day, and it will be easier if you've been sleeping well to this date.

Your stress and worry zone could be as easy as a bulletinboard or an organizer, however it is essential that this isn't brought into the bedroom. Make sure that it is a peaceful and relaxing environment! can also make use of notespads so that you can write notes to ensure that you don't need to lay in bed staring at the ceiling and looking over the items you're sure you've lost!

# Chapter 11: Changing Your Bedtime Routine

Sometimes all it takes to get sleep apnea or snoring to be gone is the change in your sleep habits. By incorporating the "rituals" listed below and adhering to these will not only help treat the problem but will improve your sleeping quality. Follow the steps and you will see the results within 30 days or shorter.

Adjust a sleeping position that is side-facing. Many people suffer from sleep apnea and snoring when they sleep on their backs (supine). In this scenario gravity causes their tongues and soft tissues that line the lower back of their throats fall. If they lie on their backs it is possible to eliminate this and prevent airway obstruction, that can panic to the snoring to stop. But, it can be difficult to maintain this position throughout the night, and eventually to adopt to this position as a habit of sleep. It is possible to test the classic technique of tennis balls:

Get a tennis ball, or any other ball that is similar in dimensions.

Attach a sock , or a pouch to the rear of your t-shirt pajama bottom by sewing it or using an safety pin.

Put the tennis ball into the socks

Alternately, you can put tennis balls in an inflatable wedge pillow, which you can place in front of your back.

The tennis ball is uncomfortable, and in time you'll be able to make side-sleeping routine and not have to use the ball as often. Another option is to put the body pillow to your back. These are pillows that are fully-length that support your whole body. There are companies that make specially-designed products, that prevent sleep supine. You may want to look for them too.

Make sure you prop your head up. By elevating your body from your to the waist using a foam wedges, or raising your head by between four and six inches will prevent forward motion of your jaw and tongue which can cause obstruction of your airways. The cervical pillow is employed for the same reason and also help prevent your neck muscles from becoming painful.

Beware of sleeping tablets, sedatives or alcohol. They can induce a more restful sleep, which relaxes the muscles of your throat which makes it harder for your airway to remain open. It's been observed that those who don't normally snore usually do so after drinking alcohol for four to five hours prior to sleeping.

Open your nasal passages. A nasal congestion can make breathing difficult but also creates an air bubble in your throat that can generations to snoring.Try to rinse your nose before bathing at night, or apply saline spray respiratory strips, a nasal dilators neti pot (salt-water solution) or allergy medicines.If your issue is located in your nose and not in the soft palate, try applying nasal strips. Speak to your doctor to find out whether these solutions can improve your situation.

Make sure the air is humid. Utilize a humidifier as dry air can trigger irritation to the throat and nose membranes. This can cause snoring.

Clean your bedroom of dust. Make sure your bedroom is clean particularly your electric fan, as dust that gets into your respiratory system could cause irritation, leading to sleepiness. It is also important to be careful not to allow pets to rest in your home since they could make you breathe in pet dander, which is another airway irritation.

Take note of what you eat. Avoid dairy products, caffeine as well as heavy meals for at least 2 hours prior to falling asleep. Caffeine can be a stimulant which can disrupt sleep and could connected in snoring. Dairy products cause mucus to build inside your airway which is the reason for snoring.

Replace your pillows. Dust mites that have accumulated within your pillows could cause allergic reactions and irritation to your airways like the effects of dust. It is suggested to put your pillows on the air fluff routine every two weeks. Also, you should change them every six months to help keep dust mites and allergens at an absolute minimal. When selecting your pillows, you could choose a pillow specially made to stop snoring make sure you test the pillows carefully if they cause discomfort, like neck discomfort.

Keep yourself hydrated. Consuming water in a regular basis can stop your nose and palate from getting sticky. This results in airway obstruction that can distinct to more sleepiness. Healthy women require a minimum eleven cups in fluid consumption (including liquids from food) per day, while men require around 16 cups.

Maintain a healthy sleep routine. If you are working all day long and hard without sleeping enough in the previous night, you're hitting the bed tired. This can have the same effect like drinking alcohol and sleeping pills, or sedatives. You get a good night's sleep, but you are also exhausted which makes your throat muscles less flexible and more likely to block your airway.

# Chapter 12: Follow A Sleep-Friendly Diet

Food is the body's source of energy. Consume high-quality foods and you'll be able to perform better. Pick low quality food items However, your body will breakdown like a battered car without fuel. It is not surprising that food can affect the quality of our sleeping.

Consider, for example the results of a study conducted in 2012 which published in The Journal of Clinical Endocrinology and Metabolism. They found that people who drink and eat foods designed to give you a brief power boost are also the ones who are progressively overweight and experience less sleep.

So, get rid of the afternoon cup of coffee and slice of sweet cake. Instead, stick to a healthy balanced diet that will boost your energy levels, cut off your waistline and ensure you a great sleep.

Here are some tips for a healthy diet to remember:

Make sure you adhere to a strict eating plan.

It is essential to eat your meals at regular time slots throughout the day as this helps your brain to adhere to a certain system. This will prompt you to go to bed and rise at the same time every day.

It's simple to create the timings of meals. For example, if you get up around 7 a.m. each day and plan to eat breakfast around 7:15. After 3 hours, you can have some light breakfast. About 12:30 p.m. take lunch, before enjoying a lunch snack at the end of three hours. Then, you can take a meal at 6:30 p.m. Also, enjoy some light snacks or a warm drink around 9:15 p.m.

Set alarms to prompt you to do this first, to build the habit. Then, you'll adhere to them more naturally.

Reduce caffeine intake.

It is possible to argue that you require coffee to perform at a high level throughout the day but the reality is, you don't need it, especially when you are following an appropriate diet. If you do decide to have coffee, be sure that you drink it in the period between 9 to 10 a.m. to ensure it won't affect your sleep later.

Limit your intake to three cups of 8-ounces of coffee, as per the National Sleep Foundation.

Remove the sugar.

Sugar is bad in terms of health. It doesn't have any nutritional value and does nothing but temporarily increase the blood sugar levels. While this might result in an energy boost however, it can lead to a crash which will cause your desire for more sugar. The addiction can withdrawal to a drastic change in levels of energy that prevent you from getting the needed rest. Even more is the risk of developing Type 2 Diabetes.

Instead, eat healthier alternatives. If you do have to have something sweet, go with an alternative that is more natural sugar like maple syrup or honey.

Consume healthy, nutritious foods that help encourage sleep

Complex carbs can be your most trusted all-rounder when it comes to sleeping. They are made up of gluten-free or whole wheat grains. It is also suggested to add a little lean protein to improve sleep further. So , grab some brown rice or whole wheat bread, and some buckwheat noodles at dinner.

Apart from complex carbohydrates You should also eat these meals throughout the day, as they're known to have certain natural elements that to promote sleep better:

Lettuce contains lactucarium

Kale-rich in calcium

Halibut and tuna are high in vitamin B6.

Shrimp and lobsters are rich in tryptophan

Dairy products that are high in calcium

Pistachio nuts are rich in vitamin B6

Walnuts are a source of tryptophan

Almonds are high in magnesium

Chickpeas high in tryptophan

Garlic is a rich source of vitamin B6

Herbal teas to aid in sleep

In the years since the invention of herbal teas that are hot many people have turned towards it for better sleep. There are a variety of options out there, here's an inventory of the plants that are the most well-known for sleeping:

Chamomile

Valerian

Lavender

Peppermint

Lemon Grass

Lemon Balm

St. John's Wort

# Chapter 13: The Causes And Comorbidity

The most common cause of insomnia is that it coexists or is a result of:

If psychoactive substances are employed, which includes stimulants that involve particular herbs, medicines like caffeine, nicotine amphetamines, cocaine modafinil, aripiprazole, methylphenidate, MDMA or increased intake of alcohol.

If the anti-anxiety medication is stopped such as pain relievers (opioids) and benzodiazepines.

Any heart disease

Thoracic surgery history

The respiratory system is prone to problems, including problems with breathing at night, and nasal septum that is deviated

Restless legs syndrome could cause slumber-onset sleep lack (sleep in the onset of insomnia) due to the uncomfortable sensations that are felt and the desire to move leg or any other part of the body in order to ease these feelings.

A disorder of the limbs called periodic limb movements (PLMD) is a condition that occurs in the midst of sleep and may cause arousals in which the sleeper is not conscious.

A nagging or painful issue that causes pain may prevent a person from locating a comfortable posture to drift off. It can be arousing.

Changes in hormones, such as the ones that occur prior to menstrual cycles and menopausal changes.

Life events, like tension, anxiety tension, emotional or mental anxiety, pressure at work financial anxiety grieving, conception, and grief.

Gastrointestinal issueslike constipation, acid reflux or constipation.

Mental illness, for instance bipolar issue and generalized anxiety disorder post-traumatic anxiety, schizophrenia, dementia obsessive-compulsive disorder and ADHD

The unsettling effects of the circadian rhythm like the effects of jet lag and motion work could cause a lack of energy to relax at various periods of the day, and excessive sluggishness at various periods during the course of the day. Chronic disorders of the circadian rhythm are represented by similar symptoms.

Certain neurological issues cerebrum trauma, an earlier history of traumatizing brain injuries.

The most common therapeutic conditions are hyperthyroidism or rheumatoidarthritis.

The use of prescription and solution-based tranquilizers (soothing or depressant drugs) can trigger bounce-back sleepiness.

Poor sleep hygiene, e.g., clamor or excessive consumption of caffeine.

A rare hereditary issue can cause a prion-based long-lasting and eventually deadly form of sleeping disorder known as the fatal family insomnia.

Physical physical activity. Sleep deprivation due to activity or insomnia is common among athletes because of the prolonged latency in onset of slumber.

Studies of sleep and rest using polysomnography have suggested that people who suffer from interruptions to their sleep have elevated levels at nighttime of the hormones cortisol as well as adrenocorticotropic. They also have an elevated metabolic rate. This isn't the case in people who don't suffer from sleep loss, yet whose sleep is disturbed in an investigation into slumber. Research into the metabolism of the brain through positron emission tomography (PET) outputs have shown that those suffering from a sleep disorder experience higher metabolic rates at night and during the daytime. It is unclear if these patterns are caused by or a result of long-term sleepiness.

Insomnia and steroid hormones

The research has led to steroids and sleep disorder. Cortisol levels fluctuate and progesterone during the female cycle or estrogen during menopausal changes can be correlated with more frequent episodes of sleep lack. Individuals with differing levels of cortisol often experience insomnia over a long period in which insomnia is caused by the an increase in estrogen caused by menopausal changes and progesterone causes the cause of insomnia in a shorter time during the monthly lapse of the women's cycle.

Cortisol

Cortisol is often regarded as the hormone that causes anxiety in humans but it's also the hormone that causes wakefulness. The analysis of salivary samples, which are that are taken at dawn and evening, has revealed that those who suffer from insomnia awake with lower levels of cortisol in comparison to those with normal sleeping patterns. More research has revealed that people with less cortisol levels after awakening have less memory contrasted with those who have normal level of cortisol. Research suggests that greater amounts of cortisol released at night is a sign of insomnia primary. For this reason, medicines that are associated with a issues with cooling state of mind or unease, like antidepressants, can control cortisol levels and in preventing insomnia.

Estrogen

Many postmenopausal women have noticed changes in their sleep routines after menopausal transition which could be a sign of insomnia-related side effects. It could be due to decrease in estrogen levels. Low estrogen levels could cause hot flashes, changes in the anxiety response or a general change in the sleep cycle which can all contribute to sleep loss. Estrogen treatment and estrogen-progesterone mix supplements as a hormone substitution treatment can help direct menopausal ladies' slumber cycle again.

## Progesterone

Progesterone levels that are low throughout the female menstrual cycle, but particularly towards the final stage of the luteal cycle are also thought to be linked to the onset of insomnia, peevishness, and irritability in females. A majority of women are suffering from sleep issues prior to or during menstrual cycles. The lower levels of progesterone may similarly as estrogen, cause menopausal women experiencing insomnia.

An underlying misconception is that the amount of sleep decreases when a person gets older. The capacity to sleep for prolonged periods rather than the need to sleep, creates the impression that you are lost as people get older. A few elderly people who are sleep-deprived or sleepy individuals toss and turn throughout the night in bed which reduces the amount of sleep they get.

## Risk factors

Everyone of any age is affected by insomnia, however those within the categories below are more likely to getting a sleep disorder.

Aged 60+ of age

The history of mental illness, including Depression, etc. on.

Anxiety and emotional stress

Night shifts that are late at night

Travelling through time zones that are different

# Chapter 14: Diagnosis Of Sleep Apnea

The method used by doctors to determine sleep apnea is based on the medical history and family history. They also conduct an physical exam. They will look at your signs. If they think that your signs, symptoms, and patterns are consistent with this condition and you're going be recommended to a sleep test.

Sleep studies are studies which reveal your sleeping patterns. The results reveal how much and how you sleep. If you are experiencing problems with your sleep these studies will to provide the results of those.

If you're referred for an investigation into your sleep it is crucial to get one. The test will determine whether you've had a diagnosis of a sleep-related disorder, such as sleep apnea. Sleep apnea, along with other sleep disorders could increase the risk of strokes, hypertension , and cardiac arrest.

The doctors who are skilled in studying sleep patterns can swiftly identify sleep apnea and provide treatments to help you rest better at night. It is essential to inform your physician of any sleeping issues you've experienced.

These could include fatigue and persistent drowsiness throughout the daytime. Also, consult your physician when you've had difficulties sleeping or waking at the end of the night and aren't able to go back to sleep.

It is possible that you have an issue with your sleep which you're not aware of. Doctors who specialize in sleep disorders will inquire about your sleeping habits. They'll also consult your family members family about any snoring issues they've had to deal with.

Doctors with experience in sleep disorders are known as specialists in sleep. They are able to quickly recognize and provide treatment for those suffering from difficulties with sleeping.

To assist experts in determining the root of the problem it is recommended to create and maintain a sleep diary not more than two weeks. This is the beginning of the study of sleep. Here are a few questions you could find in a journal of sleep:

The time you went to bed at night prior to

The time that you got up in the early morning

The amount of time you slept before going to bed

The amount of times that you were up in the middle of the night

- How was the time it took you to get to sleep for the night?

What drugs did you take in the evening prior to your sleep?

If you were awake and groggy when you got up in the morning, you'd be wide awake.

If you're drowsy at the time you woke early in the morning

- - The amount of beverages with caffeine that you consumed during the day

The quantity of alcohol you consumed during the day

The time that you consumed alcohol

The number of naps you took

The length of those napping sessions

If you're really tired throughout the day

If you're somewhat tired throughout the day, you may have been tired.

If you were alert throughout the day, you were likely to be alert.

If you were awake all day

Your doctor may also inquire about the following issues:

Snorting.

- A gasp.

Headaches in the morning.

If the findings from the journal suggest:

Regular naps.

- Then waking up a few times during the night.

Needing more than half-hour to get a good night's sleep.

Constantly feeling sleepy during the daylight.

Physical Examinations to Determine Sleep Apnea.

During your physical examination Your doctor will be examining the mouth, nose and throat. They'll be looking to locate enlarged or additional tissues. If a child is suffering from sleep apnea the majority of them have tonsils that are enlarged. In these cases, it will not require much to make a medical diagnosis other than an examination and a medical background.

For those who are older, the doctors look for an expanded uvula. It is a tissue that is located in the middle of your mouth's rear. They also search to find a soft palate which is found at the throat's back and is also known by the name of the mouth's roof in this area.

How family members can help in identifying sleep Apnea.

Because most people don't know that they're suffering from sleep apnea it's important to have someone who can detect irregularities while you rest. It is not known that their breathing may start and stop anytime during the night. They don't consider when someone says they are a an intractable and a loud snorer.

There are some things that members of the family could do to help:

• Let a member their family understand that they suffer from a long-running problem of loud snoring.

Inform them to see their physician.

In the event that they're diagnosed as having sleep apnea. advising that they follow the guidelines which include post-operative treatments, follow-ups, and follow-ups.

- Helping them emotionally. This can be a challenging moment for them and they'll need all the assistance they can receive.

# Chapter 15: Diet-Related Factors

Caffeine: It is a potent nervous system stimulant, typically present in coffee, tea as well as chocolate and sodas.

Point 1: There's a time when the body is able to settle down into a resting state after the right levels of adenosine have been attained. Coffee functions by filling receptors for the adenosine. Instead of feeling exhausted the body continues to go on since it's not getting the right signals that let it rest and recuperate.

Point 2. Caffeine's effects can be experienced by the body after 5 to 8 hours following the consumption.

Tips for a Sleep Solution:

Do not consume caffeine after 2 at o'clock in the afternoon. This will make sure that your body has eliminated it completely from its system before going to bed.

Magnesium: The mineral is believed to possess properties that reduce stress. Its sleep-related effects include relaxing muscles that are tense and relaxing your nervous system.

Point 1. Research has proven some signs of magnesium deficiency is constant insomnia, or difficulties sleeping.

2. The most effective method for raising magnesium levels within the body is by applying a treatment of this mineral to the skin.

Tips to Improve Sleep:

Include magnesium-rich foods into your diet, such as:

Green leafy vegetables

Pumpkin seeds

Sesame seeds

Spirulina

Brazil nuts

Bathing in Epsom salts can aid in the absorption through the skin of magnesium. Other types of magnesium applied to the skin are magnesium bath flake, and magnesium oils.

The best locations to apply magnesium topical are:

Anywhere on the body that is affected by pain.

On the chest

Around the neck and shoulders.

drinking alcohol late into the evening can cause a person to fall asleep quicker, but sleeping quality is greatly affected.

Point 1: When alcohol is present in the system it is not in a position to go deep levels of rest.

Point 2: One of most frequent sleep disruptions that result from drinking is the necessity to go through urine. When a person awakes from a sleep-deprived state it may be difficult to get back to sleep.

Tips to Improve Sleep:

Do not drink alcohol for at least 4 hours prior to going to sleep.

Drinking water may help reduce alcohol's effects and aid in flushing it out quicker.

Sleep-inducing supplements:

1. Chamomile It is a herb that has the capacity of helping relax the nervous system as well as in relaxing muscles.

2. Kava kava is a drink which originated from Fiji and is a sedative drink. It is commonly used to treat fatigue and insomnia. Its properties help improve sleep quality as well as reduce the amount of time required to go to sleep.

3. Valerian Valerian: This herb is a mild sedative that is suggested for those who have difficulty getting to sleep. It can also aid in achieving a peaceful sleep.

4. 5-HTP: It is a neurotransmitter, which acts as an precursor to serotonin which is involved in the your sleep. Research has shown that those who took 5-HTP were able to more quickly fall asleep and could sleep longer.

5. GABA is the most important inhibitory neurotransmitter that the brain produces and is a key factor in the process of causing sleep. It can block the action of excitatory brain chemicals and allow the brain to relax and relax.

6. L-Tryptophan is the precursor of 5-HTP that was previously mentioned. Food sources include chicken, turkey and pumpkin, sunflower seeds and collard leaves

7. Melatonin: Melatonin is effective in promoting sleep, however, the drawback is that it may affect the body's natural capacity to create Melatonin itself. Additionally, many hormonal treatments like this can cause many adverse effects and health issues.

The Side Effects of the Drug:

irritability

dizziness

migraines

constipation

stomach pain

weight gain

Tips for a Sleep Solution:

Supplements can be of the greatest benefit when utilized the shortest time frame to restore sleep patterns that were temporarily disrupted , for example when traveling.

Some Night Snacking Sleep Solution Tips:

If you are experiencing hunger pangs prior to bed, it's best to eat a fat-rich low-carbohydrate snack in order to ensure that your blood sugar remains level stable and to prevent sugar spikes that could cause sleep disruption.

At least ninety minutes after eating prior to going to bed.

# Chapter 16: Natural Remedies for Mild Disorders

There are many natural methods to deal with the issue. One of the first steps is making sure you are able to identify the problem. After determining the cause an appropriate course of action can be taken. There are several methods to deal with the issue when the diagnosis is established. In the event that the diagnose is solely OSA then the problem is specifically on the reduction of that obstruction's size. In many instances the obstruction could be congenital or may be a result of an underlying cause that causes the growth of airways' tissue. A major reason is allergy as well as the long-term consequences of allergy medication.

There are many available over-the-counter remedies to treat sleep apnea. However, If you plan to use western medications the most effective course of action should be to consult a medical professional to provide the appropriate medication.

However, if you'd prefer to find the root of your issue and solve it on your own, then this is the right chapter for you.

Remember that the first step is always to establish a correct diagnosis.

The natural remedy program starts with a strong physical foundation, which can only be achieved by a vigorous workout. Remember, we evolved from a very athletic ancestor, and we had to search for food. Our bodies are made for vigorous activity, and when this activity is not maintained and we become unhealthy. So, the first thing to ensure that you keep your body well-maintained by doing regular exercise.

If you suffer from OSA losing weight can help in curing the disease. It also helps return your body back to how it was designed to perform. A half hour of exercise one day, broken down between 20 to 20 minutes of vigorous activities as well as 40 mins of moderate activities, will enable your body to decrease fat storage, and consequently lessen the chance obstructions in the airways.

Don't sleep on your back!

Another option is to rest on one's side , not lying on one's back. If you sleep facing forward and is prone to falling asleep, there is a greater likelihood of gravity causing additional tissue to slip into the air and block it. Better to sleep on your back. When you lay on your side, particularly for those who have OSA You will experience relief since the affected tissue will be pulled downwards into the air passage. There are those who cannot sleep on their backs. In this instance you will need to determine if the left side or right side is where the issue is. If you can determine that, then it is possible to rest on the opposite side and back. In certain situations lying on the back can cause the tongue and soft palate to sit on throat's back which can cause obstruction to the airway. This is a risky scenario for those suffering from sleep apnea. Install a bolster on your back to ensure you don't roll over. When you sit onto your back, it will be extremely uncomfortable. This can be an indication to stay on your back. This can be an effective method to treat minor symptoms in Sleep Apnea.

Yoga and Meditation

In the midst of all the soft exercises I've tried and tried, the one that produces the most effect is yoga. Yoga is a great way to tone muscles and stretch the body. It also promotes peace in the body. The stretching and calming effect have a direct effect on the air passageways, and can even increase their flexibility and less blocked. Making sure your airways are free of obstruction is one of the most important factors in treating sleep apnea. The breathing exercises that are part of yoga can assist you in controlling your breathing pattern and, in turn, you will be able to overpower sleep apnea.

Additionally If you are capable of meditating and yoga, the power of yoga and meditation will increase your capacity to heal. Meditation can help you manage the intensity and the quality of your breathing by being conscious, not a routine.

Do not take sleep aids

A lot of people use sleeping pills for sleep. This can cause two issues. The first is that sleep apneics depend on their brains to awaken them when there is a breath pause. The issue of sleeping tablets is their capacity to wake up is decreased. It is the body's protection mechanism.If the patient does not awake when breathing stops, they might be suffocated.

Another issue is that these medications are in fact relaxation agents. When they really need in order to maintain their muscles awake in tightness, these tranquilizers can do the exact opposite , and may create a blockage of the airway.

Then raise your head

Then, raise your head of at least four inches from an area that supports the other parts of your head. But, this can't be accomplished by simply placing pillows underneath your neck. If done this way it will cause the head to tilt around the neck and create an airway bend that defeats the intent. The entire body should be placed on an angle. This way, the neck and the torso are on the same level. The best way to accomplish this is to buy pillows specifically designed to help support your neck, head and upper torso. Or you could raise the legs of your bed to ensure that the whole bed is inclining.

Exercises for the mouth and Throat

According to experts that exercising the throat can decrease the symptoms of apnea by up to 35-40% if they are done regularly. According to research, those who exercised regularly for three months reported less sleepiness in the day, which suggests that they had a better sleep.

Chewing might not be related to sleep apnea. However, good chewing habits will cause a change that results in an even tone of muscle throughout the neck. If you chew food on one direction, you are creating the muscles of your neck in a way that is disproportionately. This is why it is advised to alternate the two sides of your mouth while you chew.

You may also place your tongue on the palate and close your mouth when chewing. This can help increase the mobility and function of your jaw and tongue and can help relieve certain signs associated with sleep apnea.

The experts also recommend tongue exercises lasting minimum three minutes which can be done at times throughout your day. Begin by cleaning the superior and lateral tongue surfaces while your tongue is resting in your mouth on its floor. Then, you can place your tongue's tip on the palate's front while sliding the tongue inwards. Next, you need pushing your tongue up until it's in contact with the palate. Following that, you should press the back of your tongue, and then place it on the floor your mouth.

The practice of articulating vowels that are open is proven to help alleviate sleep apnea. It is recommended that you breathe through your nose and exhale out of the mouth. Perform this exercise for at minimum 3 minutes at least a few times a throughout the day. This is similar to the other workout. Some of the words with long vowel sounds that you can work on are bee fly, fly, tree, and cry.

The exercises mentioned above are able to be completed at different times throughout the day, or the sets can be performed together and repeated several times throughout the day. The way you perform it is yours to decide.

Another option to try is using your toothbrush. Begin with pressing the tongue to the floor of your mouth. Utilizing a toothbrush, scrub the sides and the top of your mouth. Repeat this process five to six times, at least three times per day, or each time after you have finished brushing your teeth.

Another exercise is to keep your tongue to the top of your mouth, and then press up. Then place it on the bottom of your mouth, and push. Repeat this process for three minutes.

Also, there is the kissing practice. There is no need for an accomplice to do this practice. It is done simply by making your lips purr like you were going the kiss of your kid. Make sure that your lips are tightly closed. After that, begin shifting your lips up to your left, then back up and shift your lips to left. Repeat in the same sequence, nine times more. Experts suggest that you repeat the same sequence at least 3 times.

Keep in mind that the exercises mentioned above should be following an appropriate and accurate diagnosis. The issue should have a discussion with your doctor or at least an experienced traditional physician who is familiar with your medical background. It is important not whether the doctor approves but more because he is aware of your medical history and is able to identify anything that might be more harmful than beneficial.

In terms of diets it is recommended to do them in conjunction with the exercises mentioned above. Our diet is what we consume. A large portion of the spices, herbs and fruits we eat provide effects that are beyond just food taste. They provide significant benefits in natural ways of curing.

Eat Raw Garlic

Garlic can do two things when it comes to aiding sleep apnea. It can first aid in reducing the size of tonsils. Additionally, it can be utilized to reduce inflammation, particularly when it affects breathing. Due to this effect garlic is a great option as a remedy at home to respiratory problems.

Simply chew on a clove to get the effect you want. Be sure to not boil it or blend it prior eating. It is essential to chew it. Use only a small amount every time, as excessive garlic could burn the lining of your mouth. The reason garlic should be chewed is due to the fact that the health benefits of garlic are only taken advantage of when it is bruised or crushed. Moreover, the spray can only be effective upon direct contact , and is only lasts for a couple of minutes. In the event that you grind it using the pestle or in a blender, then the spray disperses into the air , and then degrades to give you the strong taste of garlic, but without the advantages.

Eat Walnuts

Walnuts are among the most effective home remedies in sleep apnea. They aid in improving breathing by drying out the mucosa and muscles, and also strengthening their muscles. Integrating them into your regular diet is easy. There are plenty of options available online. It is also possible to make a smoothie with walnuts and milk for a drink before going to bed.

Essential Oils

Lavender, chamomile , and primrose are a few essential oils that help to promote sleep. Primrose oil can be utilized effectively to ease inflammation. Essential oils are also utilized as a compress , and they provide a mild sedative to assist you in sleeping, without the muscle relaxants of tranquilizers. It is possible to apply lavender oil, as an example on your temples prior to going to bed in order to get to sleep quicker.

Eucalyptus Oil

Congestion can be treated using the oil of eucalyptus. It is a sign of nasal allergies, as well as an illness such as a cold. Sleep apnea may be the result of this. If you're free of congestion, you will have greater chances of breathing easily and sleeping better. This is why the oil of eucalyptus proves beneficial for those suffering from sleep apnea. For eucalyptus oil to be used to ease congestion, mix it with boiling water and breathe in the steam.

Indian Gooseberry

Add Indian gooseberry to the water, boil it. Strain the water and drink at the beginning of your day prior to starting your day and at the end of your day. . It can be added to the water and bring it to the point of boiling. Then strain the water and drink it for a drink.

This Indian Gooseberry has been proven to be a potent remedy for allergies. Most of those suffering from OSA that is caused by allergies will find relief with this method. If however, your sleep apnea has been diagnosed as CSA and this treatment is not going to help you.

# Chapter 17: Treatments for Medical Conditions for Sleepiness (Sleeping tablets/Sleep aids)

Sleep aids or sleeping tablets are medicines that aid people who suffer from insomnia sleep better. They are referred to as hypnotics, and they are typically taken to alleviate symptoms of insomnia that are short-term as well as to reduce severe symptoms of insomnia, and also if the non-medical treatment fails to have an effect.

On the other hand medical professionals and doctors are usually reluctant to recommend insomnia tablets, or even sleep aids for their patients.As as tablets for sleeping may help with insomnia but they can't solve the root of insomnia.

Sleeping pills or sleep aids do not work for people suffering from long-term insomnia.In general, doctors will recommend these patients to a psychotherapist or sleep specialist for different treatment options.

If you're prescribed sleeping pills Your doctor will likely to prescribe the lowest dose that is possible in the shortest period, typically less than one week.Otherwise in the event that your insomnia is extreme your physician is likely to suggest taking sleeping tablets two or 3 times per week instead of once a night.

Sleep aids or sleeping tablets may also trigger side effects based on the kind dosage, dosage, and response of the individual's system.They could cause an afternoon drowsiness, or even a feeling of hangover.As as such, it's advised to take sleep aids or sleeping tablets at night before going to bed.

In some instances, especially those who are older that feel hungover, it may last for a day.Thus it is recommended to take care when driving on the next day or engage in tasks that require a lot of reaction.

Important Factors to Consider While You are taking Sleeping Tablets or sleep Aids

In the majority of cases insomnia sufferers can benefit from taking the sleeping pills or other sleep supplements for help in getting to sleep or staying asleep throughout the night or enhancing the quality of their sleep.On the other side, there are a couple of things to take into consideration when you are taking sleep tablets or sleeping aids.

1.Sleeping pills or other sleep supplements could help but only after you have tried alternative or natural treatments, but insomnia is persistent and can affect your daily routine.

2.A specific sleeping tablet could be recommended after your physician has identified the root of your insomnia.As this is the case, you must not simply take one on your own.

3.Sleeping tablets , or even sleep aids aren't substitutes for natural, healthy sleeping habits.The most effective treatment for insomnia is to develop proper sleeping practices.If you have a long-running insomnia it is recommended to continue using non-medicated or natural treatments, or a combination of non-medicated treatments and sleeping tablets.

4.If you experience intermittent insomnia, taking sleeping tablets can help.If the reason for your insomnia is an incident that is temporary, such as jet lag, then it's safe to use sleep aids.However should you notice that you experience sleep problems for more than 3 days during the week, it is recommended to consult your physician and stop taking sleep aids.

5.Prior to taking sleep tablets or other sleep aids, talk to your physician if you are experiencing psychological or health effects because of difficulty sleeping.

Certain sleeping tablets and sleep aids are only available by prescription.This is due to the fact that they could be addictive and can lead in more serious health issues in the event that the form, dosage and dosage are not appropriate for your specific insomnia issue.

Different types of sleep aids Tablets as well as Sleep Aids

Benzodiazepines

These are medications for insomnia that serve as tranquilizers capable of promoting relaxation, sleep and calmness and reducing anxiety.Benzodiazepines are usually prescribed to people with severe insomnia or extreme distress due to insomnia.

The most frequent result of benzodiazepines can be sleepiness.In the event, it may anxious to dependence or addiction and that's why doctors suggest the use of these drugs for immediate effects.

Z Medicines

These are medicines that have a short-acting effect that function in the exact manner as benzodiazepines.They are thought to be the newest kind of insomnia medication.They comprise zolpidem, Zoplicone, and zaleplon.

Zolpiden is a medication that can be used for a short time to treat insomnia that is typically given at the lowest dosage and for no more than four weeks.Some of the most frequent side effects are headaches fatigue, diarrhea sleep-related issues nausea/vomiting, dizziness and stomach pains.Its lesser-known adverse effects include double vision as well as inattention.

Zaleplon is a medically licensed drug to treat people who experience difficulty getting to sleep.It is typically recommended at the lowest dosage and is prescribed for up to two weeks.Some of the possible side consequences of Zaleplon include insomnia and dysmenorrhea, or painful menstrual cycles in women, memory issues and paraesthesia, also known as pins and needles.Less frequent adverse effects of Zaleplon are a lack or coordination as well as balance issues, changes to the sense of smell and hallucinations inattention or apathy difficulties in concentration, and dizziness.

Zopiclone is also registered medicine for insomnia, specifically designed for people who experience difficulty sleeping, being awakened in the night, or suffering from chronic insomnia.It is taken in the smallest dose and should not be taken longer than 4 weeks.The typical adverse effects of zopiclone are sleepiness dry mouth, dry eyes and a metallic taste.Less frequent negative effects associated with this drug include drowsiness nausea, headaches, vomiting and nausea.

Z medications can also check to psychiatric symptoms, including anxiety, delusions, anger and aggression, as well as hallucinations, irritability and nightmares.Once you encounter one or more of these reactions, you should stop taking these medications and talk to your physician immediately.

Antidepressants

Antidepressants are generally recommended to patients suffering from insomnia, especially in the event of a previous background or a history of depression.One one of the most commonly used antidepressants prescribed to treat insomnia is Melatonin.

Melatonin is a melatonin-based medicine that has demonstrated a reduction in symptoms of insomnia.Melatonin assists in regulating the sleep cycle , which is known by the term "circadian rhythm", given the fact that it's a naturally occurring hormone.

Circadin is one of the most well-known medicine that is made up of melatonin.It is approved to treat insomnia and is only available on prescription to those who are over 55 or above.It is specifically prescribed to treat insomnia on a temporary basis that is not longer than 3 weeks.If you have kidney or liver condition It is not recommended to use Circadin to treat insomnia.

A few of the adverse effects of Circadin are constipation, dizziness and weight loss, as well as irritability stomach pain, and migraine.

Alternative Medicines

There are a variety of alternative treatments for those who are having trouble sleeping or remaining asleep through the night.On the contrary, these drugs are not able to pass the same safety tests like other types of medications.As as a result, their effectiveness and potential side effects are not known or studied.

# Chapter 18: Environmental and Sleep

Changing Your Environment

If you're truly seeking to enhance the level of quality sleep it is highly recommended you change your environment to the more favorable. Your environment is a reflection of your interactions with others, and the triggers in your environment that impact your physical, mental and emotional state and, ultimately your sleep pattern. This chapter will cover the following areas physical environment, sound electronic, lighting and social interaction.

Physical Environment

The quality of your bed and pillows affect how well you rest, as does your capacity to sleep. It is crucial to ensure that your home is set to the correct temperature to avoid anxiety. You should try to rest in comfortable clothing, and pick bedding that is suitable for your skin.

Make your living space as cozy and appealing to the eye as you can to improve sleep quality and the quality and length of your sleep.

Lighting and Sound

Incorrect lighting or sound levels can cause sleepless states. For instance, if you're exposed to noise levels that range from 40 to 70 decibels, you reduce the ability to sleep. If you've for a long time been exposed to sounds, such as traffic noises while you're asleep and you want to eliminate these sounds, it can disturb sleep too.

Light is among the most important factors that affect our sleep cycles and it plays a role in regulating the circadian rhythms. So, before you go to sleep you should avoid any bright lights. It is crucial that throughout the day you are exposed to a significant amount of bright exposure to light. However, when you sleep you need to expose yourself to enough darkness and remove the most light possible.

## Electronics

They are totally integrated in our everyday lives. They influence your sleep patterns. Certain of your most loved devices could even hinder your ability to get the best night's sleep. Because electronics emit bright light, they can hinder the brain's ability of falling asleep. Therefore, if you're looking to go to bed, don't utilize these devices prior to going to you go to bed.

## Social Interactions

It's no secret that your interactions with others could affect the quality of your sleep and also your capacity to get to sleep. If you are a victim of anger, a fight or a shock, extreme anxiety, or a serious emotional turmoil within a matter of hours of sleeping, you may be prone to restlessness and insomnia. There are several scenarios that could disrupt your normal sleep cycle

A disagreement with a coworker or significant other could trigger extreme amounts of physiological alertness such as increased pulse, heart rate and breathing.

An unfortunate experience can cause you think and create repeated thoughts that disturb your sleep.

The stress of emotional turmoil can affect sleep due to obvious reasons.

A lot of the emotional states result from interactions with other people. For the sake of getting a healthy night's sleep, make sure to be a part of the following activities:

Engage in conflict resolution to lessen conflicts. The high levels of negative emotional arousal can disrupt sleep patterns. The negative consequences of a heated argument may last for days, and take the control of your mood as well as your thinking patterns and. In addition, it may affect relaxation abilities.

Concentrate on positive interactions. create healthy relationships that don't interfere with the bodily functions.

Positive interactions are positive and relaxing influence to the brain. The more relaxed your mental and physical situation is more easy it is to sleep.

Develop healthy strategies for coping with the disappointments of life. Through this process, you be able emotionally control and minimize the emotional impact of certain circumstances. This will help you manage your mood and to relax before going to bed.

## Chapter 19: In The Room In The Room, On The Bed

If you do not like to lie on the couch, on the ground or sleeping in a tent, magic takes place in the bedroom and on the mattress. The ambience of the room is vital since it has the potential to allow you to fall asleep more quickly and enjoy a peaceful night or help you stay awake. Imagine the way you feel when you step into the space that is messy and what a difference it makes when you walk into a space which is tidy clean, smells great, and is quiet and well-lit. The same principle is applicable to the mattress. Some of the most enjoyable nights of sleep I ever had were in hotels. The comfort that you are surrounded fresh , clean sheets, pillows that are soft with minty chocolate. You don't have to stay in hotel suites constantly or have staff on the scene to keep your bedroom fresh and clean. Here are some easy suggestions on how you can perfect your bed and room to ensure you get a better night's sleep.

Switch off the lights and attempt to sleep with no lighting in the room or in a dim light. Even a small amount of light can irritate the eyes, stimulating your mind as you're asleep. Beware of any noise. I'm not talking about white noise or music. I'm talking about noise from the street or any other source that is in the room. Use earplugs to block out the sound and wear a face mask to block light any time and anywhere you are unable to be in control of these things.

One thing I've discovered that really aids me is lighting the incense candles. There are several scents that I find beneficial however others irritate me with their smell. Choose a scent that you feel familiar with and then align your mood for the day to the scent. For instance, I like to put mandarin and lime basil in the bathroom since the citrus scent brings me a sense cleanliness. In the bedroom, I love lighting candles with scents that contain saffron and magnolia. Purchase a sturdy candle holder and then fall asleep to the glow of the candle glinting across the walls of your bedroom.

Shut off the television, computer cell phone, and all other electronic devices. If you can, create a space a sanctuary that is free of any electronic gadgets . Go traditional. Keep a few books close by to read when you cannot sleep or prefer to read while in bed. You can listen to some relaxing and soothing tunes to aid you in your efforts to relax. Perhaps even natural sounds like the sounds of forests or water. It is recommended to play them with an alarm clock that can turn off completely.

Numerous recent studies have came to the same conclusion, that it's not recommended to use electronic devices while in bed , and especially before bed. This is not only dangerous as some gadgets can cause heat and start fires, but they emit radiation which can cause harm if left for long periods of time. The light emitted by their screens can also impact our eyes, and the exuberance that is generated in the brain can be difficult to stop and makes it hard to get to sleep.

Try to rest as comfortably possible. Find the best position for your sleeping and body position. The most effective way to sleep is to ensure that your neck stays straight.Do not choose a high or low-pillow while your body is resting on the side or the back. Personally, I like adding an additional pillow between my legs since it helps my hips align with my body , and assists in relaxing my back. Even though at night I'll push the pillow towards the side of my bed, it helps me fall asleep quicker.

I myself like sleeping naked at times, particularly in summer when the temperatures are hot. Although some people are unable to asleep in their pajamas, others think we're more at ease in our sleep if we're naked. If you're sharing a bed with someone else and they're happy with the idea to sleep naked, you can do it with each with each other. The contact with the skin is relaxing as well as relaxing to many and that gentle touch of someone else allows you to feel secure and secure. It's also sexy and a little asleep.

Discover the most relaxing place to sleep, and invest in comfy nightwear that isn't too loose or tight. In tight clothes, you to feel sucked in and block blood flowing freely to your legs and arms. Sleepwear that is loose can get caught in the sheets of your bed or knot itself, and may cause your partner to feel uncomfortable.

Be aware of that the temperature of your room. The most effective temperature for you to fall asleep is 65 degrees Fahrenheit which is around 18 ° Celsius. If your home has an air conditioner, or you have a heater, you can adjust the settings to maintain the temperature of your room constant. The sleepwear you wear is another important element, and I generally wear silk in the summer, and cotton in the winter.

Purchase high-quality bed sheets and a comfy mattress. It is estimated that you spend eight hours a day in bed, or one third of your time and so why not invest a good amount of money in your mattress? There's a wide range of beds to pick from and the price range is wide. You should narrow your options based on the weight capacity, other features, the price of your budget, and features which are essential to you. A quality mattress should provide a balanced balance between the firmness and bounce. It should be firm to provide your body the proper support. They also tend to last for longer. A mattress that is stiff could result in skin damage as well as sore hips and shoulders and hips, while mattresses that aren't sufficiently firm can result in back discomfort. Do not be concerned about spending an extra amount for a mattress that offers an extended lifespan and good back support. It's worthy of it!

Take into consideration the type of cloth that you buy for your bedding sheets and sleepwear. Choose fabrics that are comfortable for you and that there is no allergic reaction. Choose fabrics that don't collect dust and are easy to clean. Make sure to wash your bed sheets and pajamas often to give you the energy and confidence when you see your bed clean prior to getting ready to go to bed. Also, sprinkle chocolate mints on top of your pillows for a little extra zing of indulgence.

## Chapter 20: Entering The Sleep Mindset

In the wake of examining sleeping disorders during the previous chapter, you have the chance to look into the other factors that could be impacting your ability to rest well. It is possible that, even if have a medical issue, or exhibit some indications of some of the conditions mentioned earlier, you'll nonetheless be able to accomplish improvements by making sure that you're as prepared to be trying to fall asleep and to stay in bed for the right length of time.

In certain ways, the experience you've taken by studying this book suggests that you are ready to change your lifestyle. We've already talked about understanding your body and mind, however, it's not a bad idea to stress how crucial it is to know what situations you're in when you feel completely rested. This may appear to be a nuisance however your physical makeup demands that you rest every day, which means that you've got plenty of material to experiment with! When you're more conscious of what you need then the next step is to create a mental picture in which you will make a change This means ensuring you're in the best mental condition that you are able to be so that sleep comes more naturally and effortlessly. are going to look at solutions that can be implemented later however, in the meantime, are capable of taking some time to think of three or two things you can do to try to get more sleep or enjoy a better night's sleep.

It is likely that you have thought "well I'm just going to go to bed earlier" It could occur, however there is a chance that you've been telling yourself this the majority of nights, you discover that you are still awake even though you're asleep! Don't get too harsh on yourself. We all do it . We think that we deserve a little bit of time to yourself, or a new episode from that cult television set. We've been rewarded after having a long day, don't you think? It's acceptable from time to time but if it is becoming a routine, then you could be in trouble with your hands.

Perhaps you've thought that you must really avoid looking at electronic devices prior to you fall asleep Perhaps you have heard of the particular sort of light that comes from thesedevices, and how this could affect certain people on the speed at which they get to sleep as well as the kind of sleep they enjoy. There's certainly some truth to this idea which is not the least because of the idea that staring at these high-intensity devices late at night, especially at night, could affect your body's clock, maybe causing a delay in the beginning of sleep. Of course, there is there is a risk that these devices could impact vision, but that's an entirely different discussion. Mobile phones and tablets could, in turn influence your sleep. "It is very difficult" I hear you say.

Yes, it is true - the devices of this kind are all the rage these days It's so easy to see the status of the feeds on your social networks that you would not wish to be the last to be aware of what's happening, or for an interaction with a acquaintance to be lost. For younger generations it's the way things have been for a long time - they've grew up being aware of a world in which such devices weren't an everyday thing but that doesn't necessarily mean they aren't having an impact. For older generations the devices are not new. Perhaps they were used to reading a magazine or book in bed prior to going to sleep, or maybe later, they began to watch television before going to go to sleep, either in a different room as well in the bedroom. Screens of all kinds will likely to cause an impact, but it is the kind of light that comes from tablets and smartphones that are believed to have the most influence.

You're sure to know what's to come...

In order to put yourself in a state of mind that is more conducive to falling asleep and sleeping soundly you should try to adopt an arrangement where you're not connected to your mobile or tablet while you sleep. You can begin to slowly get rid of it by turning off your devices before you go to bed or at the very least, making sure that alerts and flashing lights are on . Flashing lights can be extremely bright during the night! This means that you'll be switching to check your feeds prior to when you sleep to checking them prior to when you sleep before turning off the device. In the future, you could finalizing your feeds just before you wash your teeth and make your bed and, even more importantly, be the last time you check things prior to heading to bed. This may sound very rigid however it's all about ensuring that your mind is relaxed as you attempt to get to sleep. If that's the case, you're much more likely to be able to fall asleep quickly and then go through all of the phases of sleep we discussed earlier.

There is no way to say you should lie down and gaze at the ceiling while you sleep, but what was the last time you grabbed a book to read at night? Give the idea a shot!

A healthy mind and body can modify to a great night's sleep. Although we might be able to manage the effects of technology and other devices however, you should think about other activities that will make you feel better. Could it be that exercising at night gets rid of a feeling of fatigue and helps you get your mind off the sand You could be able to do this by stepping outside for a couple of minutes or even a short walk through the neighborhood, the streets or in the garden. Try to see if are able to see the stars or the phases of the moon. The latter is important to know for different reasons, not the least in the event that you want absolute darkness when you sleep. A full moon can be quite shining!

A calm and peaceful mental state is likely to generations to a peaceful body ready to go to sleeping, and a restful night's sleep. Consider your preferred method of calming yourself maybe a bath in the bath, taking a shower, or listening to soft music? Be careful not to overdo it; you must go with your own preferences There are many alternatives to consider, so take a look in your sleep routine.

# Chapter 21: Sleep Apnea And Surgery

The option of undergoing a surgical procedure for Sleep Apnea may seem like an easy fix but it is important to consider the risks as well. If someone is experiencing health issues such as diabetes, hypertension, or heart problems, surgery will only be done after an analysis of the risk that these illnesses could create. The decision to perform surgery cannot be made in a single day.

The surgeon might require some time to study these aspects and determine whether it is appropriate for you to go through surgery. This is crucial when surgery on children who are small.

A surgical procedure to treat Sleep Apnea issues should only be considered once you've exhausted all other options to treat it. It could also mean you will need to remove the adenolds or tonsils. Before you go to surgery the following tests will require the intervention of your physician.

Testing for other conditions (blood pressure, heart disease, blood sugar)

X-ray

CT Scan

Blood test

The types of surgery available for sleep Apnea issues

A) Nasal Surgery

Nasal congestion that is chronic is one of the most common reasons patients are able to undergo surgery. Nasal obstructions can affect the septum, the turbinate, and the nasal tract which can further increase Sleep Apnea issues. If you've tried everything to get rid of your nasal congestion that has been bothering you for years and it's not working to resolve the issue, you may be able to think about getting nasal surgery.

The procedure of reducing the size of the turbinate is usually done in these instances and is well-received by the majority of people. It is less risky than other procedures. Once the procedure is completed is able to clear the airway and allow for better airflow.

If you suffer from a collapse of the valve due to a weak lower nasal cartilage septum can be placed to enhance the strength of the valve.

The procedures are able to be completed with ease and the patient is likely to heal quickly.

B) Soft Palate Implants

The Soft Palate implants are called "pillar procedures" which can be utilized in treating Sleep Apnea problems. It is widely utilized today and can be completed in a matter of minutes. This procedure requires the placement of three rods of polyester in the soft palate. They trigger the inflammatory response that occurs in soft tissue surrounding it.

The tissues could be strengthened This will reduce the contact with the wall of the pharynx behind and eventually reduce the risk of Sleep Apnea. The procedure is so easy that it is able to be carried out by your physician using or with no anesthesia.

c) Tongue enhancement surgery

The tongue's genioglossus muscle are strengthened in order to stop the tongue from reclining forwards when the patient is asleep. This procedure involves making small cut into the jaw boneand then removing the bone and reattaching it using a small titanium disc that can stop the tongue from slipping forward.

It's a lengthy procedure and involves a variety of modern techniques. The patient will need to be admitted for a minimum of 24-hours in the hospital and then under observation for several hours after the operation. Some doctors apply this procedure only when there is a Sleep Apnea problem is severe in a patient.

D) Lower base of the tongue reduction

The lower portion of the tongue is believed to be among the causes why sufferers of Sleep Apnea experience aggravated symptoms. The reduction of the tongue's base can be performed using a variety of advanced techniques to fix Apnea problems for patients. Radio frequency wave techniques is the most preferred method by doctorssince it has demonstrated positive results for patients, far better than many other surgeries.

It directs radio frequency waves into specific areas of the tongue without harming the surrounding tissue. This procedure is not very long and patients can be discharged within one day after the operation. An general anesthesia can be sufficient for a person to bear the discomfort during the procedure.

E) Jaw improvement

Smaller or narrower jaws may limit airflow and affect Sleep Apnea patients to a greater extent. The procedure of Maxillomandibular enhancement is recommended for the case of these patients. It can assist in improving the

171

airway by stretching and extending the frame of your jaw. To accomplish this it is necessary that the lower and upper jaw bones are equipped with titanium plates after cutting a precise hole in these jaw bones.

This is a difficult procedure that is best performed by a specialist. It is essential to choose the correct surgeon, since the procedure is extremely complex. It's also a uncomfortable procedure, which requires the patient fully sedated throughout the procedure.

The patient is expected to remain at the facility for a period of 24 to 48 hours following the procedure and will only be released once they have fully recovered. The teeth must be secured with wires and only liquid foods can be eaten to avoid pressing upon the jaws.

f) Tracheotomy

Tracheotomy surgery is used to create an opening in an individual's neck which allows for a straight path into the trachea. This kind of procedure is only available to patients who are critically sick or in emergency situations. There is the possibility of serious complications arising which could make things more complicated. It is, however, an extremely effective procedure that will eliminate this Sleep Apnea problem in a patient quickly and completely. There are a few negative side effects that can be experienced by patients after surgery. The following list of symptoms are:

If the surgery is not done properly the corrective surgery could be necessary to correct the airway or larynx.

In certain people the procedure may trigger various allergies, or even cause an infection.

If the procedure is performed incorrectly, it could connected to the scarring in the airway.

Although it's rare the tracheotomy procedure can result in a large loss of blood and may require a transfusion of blood.

The throat can be painful for a time after surgery, which makes the swallowing process difficult. food solids. However, this issue usually is gone within a few days its own.

g) Hyoid Enhancement Surgery

Hyoid suspension is a great treatment to treat Sleep Apnea. The procedure is designed to relieve Apnea problems by opening up the airway that is blocked. It requires a tiny suture is placed below the chin to help the tongue. The hyoid bone can be found within the tongue, in the area where the pharynx and tongue muscles are joined.

Since the tongue can be found to fall forward while sleeping and sleep, it can come into contact with the pharynx's wall and can disrupt airflow. The procedure requires two cuts to be made around the neck. The procedure can be completed within a couple of minutes, and the patient is discharged in a matter of minutes. There are rarely any side effects or discomfort after surgery. Since it aids in recovering quicker, more people are more comfortable with this type of procedure.

# Chapter 22: Sleep Disorders

There are many sleep disorders that could be operating as a team or independently to disturb your sleep patterns. Here are the most well-known ones:

Insomnia

Insomnia is among the top commonly encountered sleep disorder in the world and, as such, it must be addressed in deep.

Have you attempted to go into bed, with the intent of sleeping, but only to be gazing up at your ceiling for long hours? Then, you test a few of the usual methods of bringing back sleep such as reading a novel but it all goes in the ground in When you do finally fall asleep in, it's not very refreshing and you'll often awake feeling tired? Even if you answered yes, then you might have insomnia.

Sleeping disorders are a frequent issue especially in our modern society where sleep patterns are deliberately controlled to allow you to have more time at work, with colleagues or be "productive". This is a complete list of symptoms and signs that are associated with insomnia:

The gang is rooling straight at the end of the evening

If you have trouble sleeping,

- Sleeping late, and waking very early.

- Unrestful even after having slept the prescribed amount

Feeling tired throughout the day.

Appetit loss,

- Nausea,

A tonne of anxiety and depression hours

- Trouble focusing on daily problems

Frequent headaches,

- Greater error percentage in work,

Based on patterns of frequency There are 3 kinds of insomnia.

Acute Insomnia: Also called stress-induced insomnia, acute sleeplessness happens when the difficulties that keep you awake in the night or disturb your sleep last for less then 30 days. This kind of insomnia is typically caused due to a stressful work routine.

Chronic Insomnia: In contrast to chronic insomnia, acute insomnia can last for more than a year. Longer durations have extensive impacts on one's lifestyle and, consequently chronic insomnia can harm the person physically and psychologically.

Transient Insomnia is among the most commonly reported types of insomnia . It can be caused by things like travel to different time zones, the typical duration is less than an entire week.

Sleep deprivation can have a significant impact on your daily life and work. Your health will be affected as well. The effects include:

- Decreased cognitive abilities,

Work performance is reduced,

A higher risk of accidents

- Lagged reaction time

A lack of maturity in the immune system

- Obesity,

Risk of developing high-risk diseases

Disturbance in the social life,

Sleep Apnea

Also known as sleep-disordered breath, sleep apnea is defined as short, shallow breaths. It is a result from obstruction in the upper airway as the soft tissue of the throat is collapsed, either in part or completely. The blockage only lasts for short periods of time and typically lasts between 10 and 120 minutes. However, these episodes could repeat 20-30 times during a sleep hour.

Sleep apnea is a condition that causes the flow of air between your mouth and lungs isn't enough even though breathing is still. Due to these conditions, the quantity that oxygen is present in the blood could decrease. It triggers an alarm in your brain, causing you to awake just enough that the muscles of your airways are in their normal positions. Your body will then return to normal. However, the shock triggered by the sudden trigger disrupts your sleep cycle and restarts the stage you were at.

It is well-known that those who suffer from sleep apnea have a loud snore, however this is not the case all the time. Due to the frequent interruptions, and the switchover between deep and lighter sleep, the mind rarely is able to rest in a restful sleep. The next day, a feeling of anxiety and mood swings can be felt all around you.

Certain factors could increase the risk of being afflicted by Sleep Apnea.

Your tongue and throat muscles are more relaxed than they should.

Adenoids and tonsils that have been enlarged,

The head and neck shape that allows for a smaller passageway inside the mouth.

- Obesity,

- Congestion due to allergies,

Restless Legs Syndrome

RLS is a numb sensation in the legs which may cause moderate to extreme irritation as well as in a lack of sleep. People suffering from RLS always feel the necessity to walk their legs in order to alleviate the sensation and consequently are unable to go to bed. The one or both legs can be affected by this.

RLS is not solely a result of the time you're trying to fall asleep, however it can occur at periods of prolonged idleness. While you sleep, RLS is characterized by intermittent leg movements, which last from 5 to 90 seconds. Sometimes, the motion may be so intense, you could get up.

# Conclusion

I hope this book is useful in helping you know how to manage sleep disorders naturally using this guide.

Next step, apply lessons you have learned from the book and apply the step-by-step guideline in this book. You should foremost, you must change your routine and eat well, as well as reduce stress and overcome sleep disorders forever.

Thank you for your kind words and best wishes!